# Belly Dancing for fitness

# Belly Dancing for fitness

## The Ultimate Dance Workout That Unleashes Your Creative Spirit

Tamalyn Dallal

with Richard Harris

Photography by Denise Marino

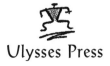

Ulysses Press

Published by: Ulysses Press
P.O. Box 3440
Berkeley, CA 94703
www.ulyssespress.com

Library of Congress Control Number: 2004101020
ISBN 1-56975-410-1

Printed in Canada by Transcontinental Printing
10 9 8 7 6 5 4 3 2 1

Managing Editor: Claire Chun
Copy Editor: Lily Chou
Editorial and production staff: Samantha Glorioso, James Meetze,
    Kaori Takee, Leona Benten
Design: Sarah Levin
Photography: Denise Marino
Movement models: Tamalyn Dallal, Jackie Lalita, Ana Sotomayor

*model credits parts 1–3: Tamalyn Dallal except on p. 10 Angela Lambru; pp 12, 16 Ana Sotomayor; p. 13 Shahar; p. 18 Montserrate Sarsotto; p. 23 Joe Zeytoonian, Tony Tahan, and Myriam Eli; p. 24 Joe Zeytoonian (on drums); pp 28, 30 Bocenka; p. 33 Feiruz.*

Distributed in the United States by Publishers Group West
and in Canada by Raincoast Books

# Table of contents

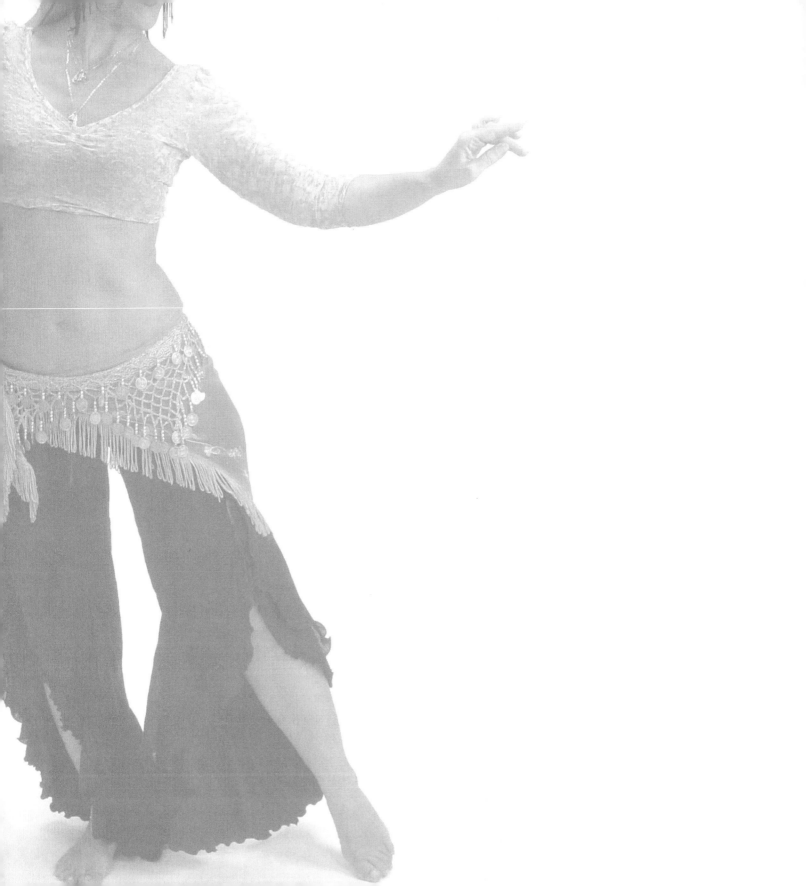

# getting started

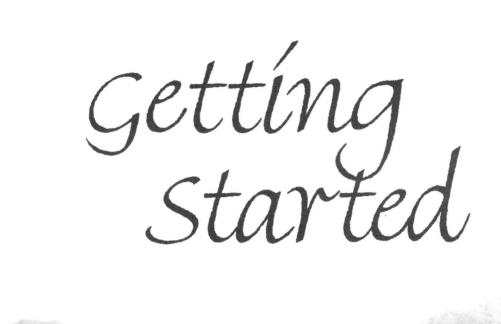

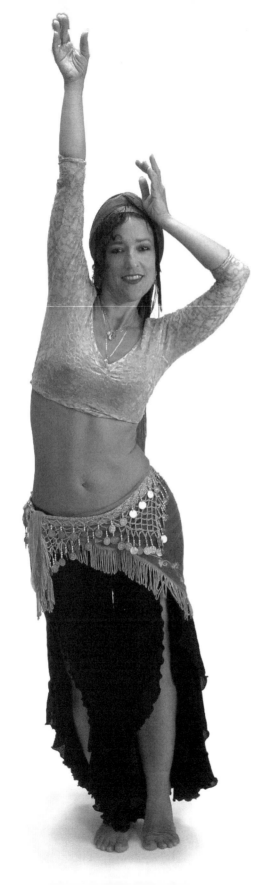

# Introduction

*W*elcome to my book—and my world. I want to share with you the basic principles of belly dancing, an art form that will burn fat and condition your abs, hips, buns, thighs, and arms as well as any conventional aerobic exercise program or TV infomercial workout machine I've ever heard of. Belly dancing will also enhance your femininity and inner beauty as it adds a new dimension of artistic creativity and spontaneity to your daily routine.

Belly dancing can also open a doorway to a wider world that is exciting, exotic, and—yes—magical. I'm not talking about the make-believe, *djinn*-in-a-lamp kind of magic, either. Belly dancing is the kind of real-life magic that can transform the way you see the world and the world sees you.

Let me start by telling you what it's done for me. Dance began to seduce me in high school. At parties, when everyone else made a beeline for the living room where rock and roll was blasting, I hung out in back rooms with the foreign students. I found their music contagious, the movements that expressed it challenging. One gathering so intrigued me that I practiced hip circles and shoulder shimmies for months, and the next thing I knew, I was on my way to becoming a full-fledged belly dancer.

I was especially drawn to Middle Eastern dance because of the costumes. My parents tell me I was obsessed with clothes from age three. By age nine, I was designing my own clothes. Belly dance presented the opportunity to adorn myself with fringe, sequins, dangling gold coins, and arm bracelets, to swirl in yards of silk veils, to deck myself out in colorful, elegant raiment one could never wear on the street—not in Seattle, anyway.

After a year of practicing the same dance movements you'll learn in this book, I took a summer job bussing tables at a Middle Eastern restaurant. Although I was too young to be allowed upstairs where they held the belly dance performances, I was able to sneak peeks at some of the famous dancers, with names like Dahlena and Badawia, who graced their stage and to hear my first full Arabic band. The owner thought I showed potential, or at least a lot of enthusiasm, and gave me a stage name: Dalal, which, I was told, meant "spoiled." I thought that was kind of rude, but every time I mentioned my new name to an Arabic speaker, they smiled fondly, remembering a sister or cousin with that name. A kinder translation, I learned, might be "pampered." I later changed the spelling to Dallal and eventually adopted it as my surname. The name has stuck ever since and has brought me a lot of luck.

From my earliest days as a dance student, I fantasized about visiting exotic places. For a while I bounced from one university to another, studying Farsi, Arabic, French, Sinhalese, Russian, and Japanese. A stint in VISTA (Volunteers in Service to America) took me to Miami, where I worked with Cuban refugees and discovered my spiritual home—an intensely multicultural city alive with tropical music, foreign languages, and romantic dark-eyed men. There I found myself passing out food stamps in a dismally bureaucratic office—until the day an opera singer friend urged, "Tami, you belong on the stage."

"But I'm saving my money so I can travel," I said.

"Performers travel more than office workers. You should consider taking your dancing to a professional level. Listen, I've traveled all over the world. How do you think I paid for it?"

"How did you?"

"My voice bought my tickets for me," she said.

Even though I couldn't sing a note, her words spoke to my soul. Sooner than you might think, right after I saw the movie *Romancing the Stone*, I was on a plane to Bogotá, Colombia. I brought along a sword, four costumes, and twenty dollars, and I danced my way around South America for the next year.

That was 21 amazing years ago. Since then, my dance career has taken me to more than 30 countries on five continents. I've been crowned Ms. America of Belly Dance and Ms. World of Belly Dance, as have two of my protegées after me. I was also one of Ark 21 Records' original "Bellydance Superstars." I've established a dance studio in South Beach, as well as a Middle Eastern dance company and a dancers'

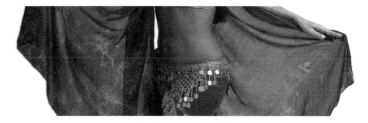

boutique. I've danced for Robert De Niro, Sean Connery, and Madonna, among many other notables. I've produced videos, live shows, and a TV series about belly dancing. I continue to work as an instructor, performer, choreographer, and producer in many parts of the world, and I plan to do so for many years to come. Best of all, I've lived the kind of adventures most women only dream about. And to think it all started with a few hip circles and shoulder shimmies!

Read on, and I'll show you how . . .

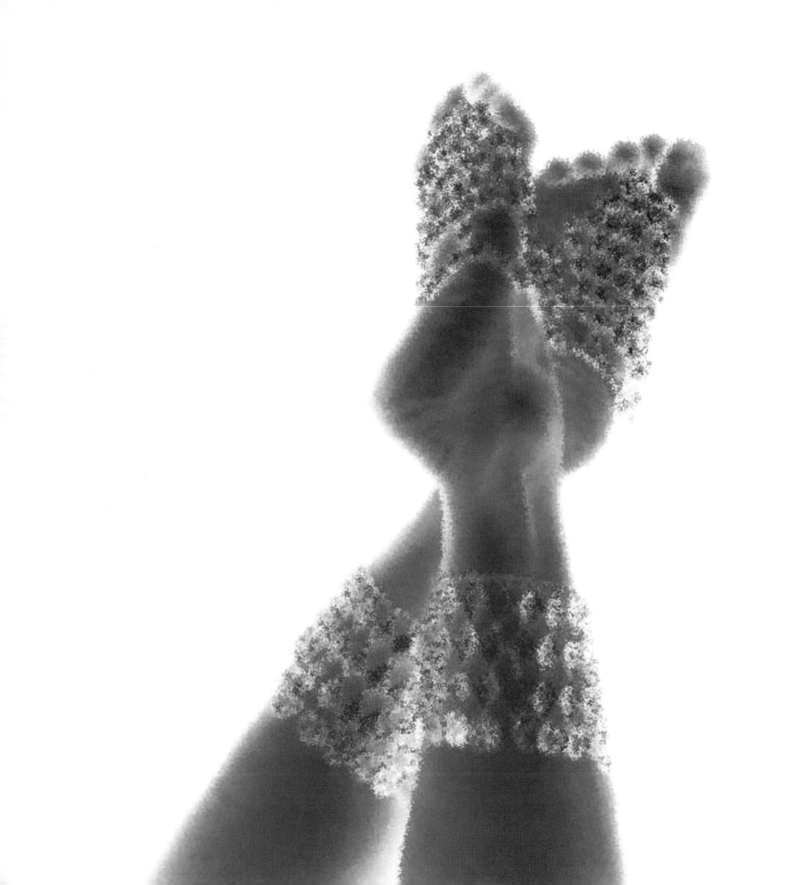

# how to use this book

*t*his book presents an easy-to-follow plan for daily belly dance workouts. If you follow the plan for eight weeks, you will experience a dramatic transformation in your physical, mental, and spiritual well-being.

In these pages you'll learn about the basic movements of belly dance, with complete instructions for doing each of them yourself. But don't make the mistake of thinking that a belly dance workout is like other, more monotonous fitness methods such as aerobics. The essence of belly dance is combining the basic movements into spontaneous, creative dance routines. This book suggests some combinations to show you how it works, but after you've mastered the basics, you can (and should) let your imagination flow. You can derive exceptional fitness benefits without ever doing the exact same routine twice.

I strongly urge you to find a local instructor and sign up for belly dance lessons. It will help a lot in learning how to do the basic movements correctly. Then you can use this book to guide you through daily practice sessions between lessons. But even if this book is your only resource—let's say you live someplace where there are no belly dance teachers, such as a small town in Alaska—you can use it to learn and practice these movements, put them together to create your own belly dance routines, and have a lot of fun getting more and more physically fit.

In addition to the movements, you'll find knowledge and insights to help your interest in belly dancing grow, such as tips on costumes and performing, a little about belly dance's rich history, and insights into Middle Eastern music. There's also a list of resources, including instructional videos, publications, and websites.

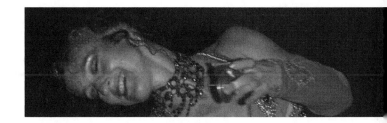

*The world doesn't need any more Hummers, leather shoes, or new flavors of chips, but it definitely needs more belly dancers.*

— a man named John
on an airplane

# Is belly dancing for you?

You never know until you try. It is a dance for women of all ages. Some start as children, others as middle-aged or older women. There is no age limit, nor is there any special body type. Belly dancers are tall, short, heavy, or thin. There is such a myriad of movements and ways to express yourself that everyone can discover her own niche.

Belly dance is about accepting your natural body type. If you are rounded and soft, why waste your precious life force trying to get buns of steel? Appreciate the fact that you have something to shimmy, and enjoy it.

Use your individuality and don't try to be like models, athletes, or even popular Egyptian dancers. Be yourself. Accept yourself. Find the beauty in your individuality and make the most of it!

## Can Men Belly Dance?

The movements in belly dance are distinctly feminine. In the Middle East, many men have become excellent teachers and choreographers, but they rarely perform belly dance in public.

At times in history, young men have danced professionally in coffeehouses, covered up and disguised as women because women were not allowed to perform in public. You can still see this in Morocco, where men occasionally dance in women's *shikhat* (entertainer) clothing.

In the United States and Europe, some men have been bitten by the belly dance bug, creating their own style of costuming and movements and becoming successful belly dance artists in their own right.

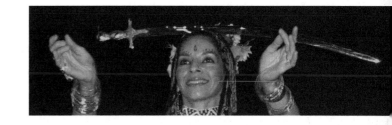

*There is no reason why belly dancing, one of the rare art forms created and conceived by women, cannot embrace men into its fold.*

# health & fitness benefits

Belly dancing is one of the world's oldest forms of exercise. A dance and exercise discipline created by women for women, it gradually evolved over thousands of years to tone a woman's body from the inside out.

## Cardiovascular and Muscular Benefits

The fast movements, primarily the hip and shoulder shimmies, offer cardiovascular benefits and make you break a sweat. The entire body is strengthened by using movements with one hip, keeping the weight on one leg. Lifting the arms for "Snake Arms" strengthens them, and many of the torso movements make the stomach strong as well as flexible.

One of the most important health benefits is that, when done with the correct posture, belly dancing stretches and releases tension in the back and strengthens the muscles, so a belly dance student who practices regularly is less likely to develop back problems. Some students complain that their backs hurt when they practice at home, and when I check their posture, their hips are usually too far forward and their chest slouched back, or vice versa. The hips are arched back when, instead, the stomach should be pulled in and the spine straight, chest forward (see "The Importance of Posture," page 36).

Students with arthritis in their hands or shoulders have told me that the gentle circular motions of belly dancing helped relieve a lot of the stiffness and pain. If you're one of those people who find it hard to stick to a program of aerobics, calisthenics, or jogging, belly dance may be the ideal fitness method for you. First, it's low-impact, meaning it doesn't jolt or jar your body and cause sore joints, a major source of discouragement for beginners in other kinds of exercise plans. Second, it emphasizes creativity and spontaneity, not mere boring repetition, so anyone who has the soul of an artist may forget that she's exercising at all and simply flow with the sheer joy of it.

## Relaxation and Stress Reduction

Belly dancing relaxes the mind as well as the body since it calls for relaxation and focus, like meditation in motion. The concentration on relaxing and isolating individual parts of the body, while losing yourself in hypnotic Middle Eastern music, has both mental and physical benefits, and these—along with the spiritual aspects of our being—are intertwined.

Many stress-related conditions can improve with the dance. One of my students who had been plagued by migraines for years told me that every time she gets a migraine, she puts on her belly dance music to practice, and it helps a lot. My own personal experience is that when I feel anxious or upset, I can teach or take a belly dance class, or do at least half an hour of practice (with music), and the scope of my problems seems to shrink into a more manageable context by the time I take a rest.

## Internal Massage

It is often said that the belly dance originated as preparation for childbirth. In the past 2000 years or so, belly dance has come a long way in terms of both artistry and fitness. In any case, belly dance certainly helps women by massaging the internal organs. Some dance students report that their menstrual cramps improve when they belly dance. Many claim that practicing the dance for at least a year before becoming pregnant helped their muscles prepare for an easier childbirth. Of course, to achieve these benefits, you have to use your belly when you dance (see "Arch/Contraction," pages 48, 49).

## weight control and Self-Image

I especially recommend belly dancing for women and teenagers with eating disorders. I can attest that many years ago, it helped me completely overcome anorexia. On the other hand, belly dancing is also effective for weight control, not only burning calories but also raising the metabolic rate to keep lost fat from coming back. Many women find it especially helpful for getting back into shape after childbirth.

However, if you get into belly dancing for weight loss, you may well discover that the real problem was not weight but self-image. Despite what the media may tell you, beauty does not depend on body type but on your awareness of your own femininity, as reflected in your posture, grace, body language, facial expressions, and glow of good health. Ask any man. (And if he tells you beauty does depend on the configuration of your body, maybe it's time to keep an eye out for another man.)

Since belly dancing embraces all body types, it relieves some of the pressure that is heaped on Western women from the first time they open a fashion magazine. In a belly dance class, the most glamourous fashion model can dance beside a voluptuous middle-aged woman—and if the model is stiff or awkward, and Ms. V. knows how to move with grace and fluidity, guess where the onlooker's eye gravitates to. Movement speaks, and it supercedes the superficial values placed on us through advertising and media bombardment.

I have seen many women change and become more beautiful after they start belly dancing. Their self-confidence improves, their posture changes, they carry themselves better and radiate a different glow. The exercise of belly dance stretches us, makes us sweat and smile at the same time, and so improves muscle and skin tone. Belly dance also inspires women to acknowledge, express, and celebrate their femininity, which makes them want to dress with a little more sizzle, or even show a little bit of

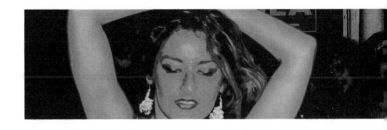

belly that they finally realize is beautiful and natural—not something to be ashamed of and try futilely to change by spending thousands of dollars on liposuction and diets.

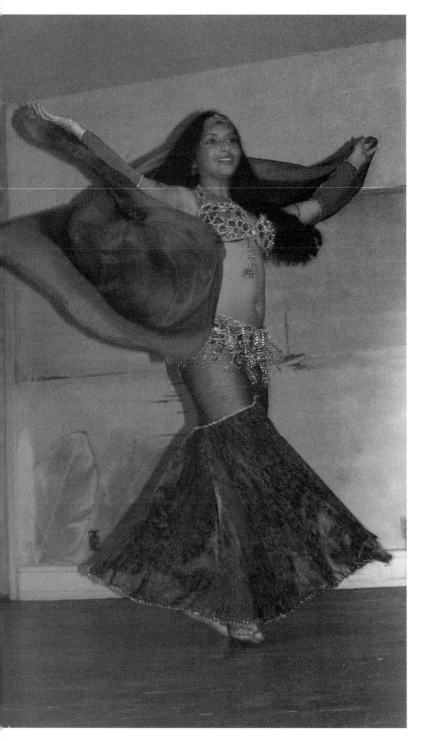

# getting ready

## workout wear

When you dance, the first priority is comfort: your clothes should be stretchy and not constricting. Some people want to come to class in jeans or street clothes, but these do not allow for proper movement.

Go to a dance supply shop and buy either a **leotard** (if you don't want to show your stomach) or a short top that stretches, such as a **sports bra or workout top** that bares your midriff.

You should also invest in some stretchy **leggings or jazz pants**. I prefer those that are fitted rather than loose because they show the movements of your legs. Though the legs should remain a mystery while you are performing, they are an important part of the dance. With your feet and legs, you control you hips, so your workout wear should let you see in a mirror what they are doing. Some people wear shorts, but since you are going to shimmy, it is best to wear your leggings either just below the knee or full length. A **long skirt** is also acceptable. Though skirts do not show your legs, they have the benefit of making you feel feminine, which helps you dance better.

The third item you will need is a **hip scarf**. They come in many varieties. Those from Egypt have elaborate hand beading, coins, or both. (A list of vendors and websites where you can purchase them is in the back of this book.) Many teachers also sell the scarves to their students, and shops that carry belly dance supplies are popping up in most large cities. Turkey produces a different style of hip scarf, which is becoming popular in the United States as well; these scarves are shinier. Be careful about the quality and take a good look at the workmanship before you buy them. There are also nice crochet and sequin shawls made in China. These are very popular in belly dance classes because they are both lightweight and pretty.

Since belly dance is the most feminine art form, you will connect much better to the dance if you dress feminine as well. Instead of a T-shirt and baggy pants or sporty-looking clothes, I recommend getting in the mood with a more sensual, exotic look. See if you have some dangly earrings, or some jewelry with coins. Let your hair hang loose, and maybe add a little lipstick or smoky eye makeup. A flower or some sparkles in your hair never hurts. Have fun!

## Shoes

The most sensuous way to belly dance is barefoot. If you have delicate feet or are not comfortable with the surface where you are practicing belly dance, you can use ballet slippers, Hermes sandals, or flat jazz shoes with a smooth sole. No sneakers, please. Also, it is best not to dance wearing socks or stockings because they can be too slippery.

## Your Workout Area

For belly dance workouts or practice sessions at home, the first consideration is to use a spacious area where you can move freely without risk of crashing into anything. It's true that belly dancers are sometimes called upon to perform in close surroundings such as restaurants or parties with limited space. But the more cramped the space, the more skill it takes to dance there, and the more restricted your choice of movements will be.

A living room or family room can be a good dance space. Make sure to remove any low furniture like ottomans or coffee tables that you could run into, and be aware of any items on shelves, mantels, or other surfaces that you could knock off with an arm movement. If you're really into it, a spare bedroom with little or no furniture in it can be converted into a great person-

al dance studio/exercise room. Even a basement can work, at least in warm weather, though you may find that dancing barefoot on a cold concrete or tile floor dampens your enthusiasm.

The ideal floor surface is hardwood or plywood finished with varnish or clear polyurethane. Most dance studios use a wood floor that is "sprung"—that is, one that is laid over crisscrossed beams so it has air underneath. But for workouts and practice sessions at home, just about any even surface, including

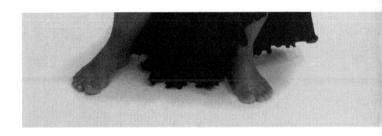

a carpeted floor, will do. Don't dance where there are loose rugs you could trip on or other hazards like children's toys or slippery wet spots.

When practicing belly dance on your own, it's most helpful to have a mirror where you can watch yourself and check your posture against the photos in this book. Many belly dance studios have a whole wall covered with mirror panels. This may not fit in with your home decor (though it sure does make the room look huge), but at least hang a full-length mirror on your wall or door where you can watch yourself practice.

Some kind of sound system is essential, of course. Most performing dancers prefer a portable boom box CD player that can be carried around to parties as a backup in case the hosts' sound system conks out. Also, if you want to use belly dance instruction videos, you can set up a TV with a videocassette or DVD player in your workout area. If you have one, you might even think about setting up a video camera so that you can record yourself dancing and watch it afterward.

Finally, some belly dance photos or Middle Eastern decor on the walls can provide a little extra inspiration.

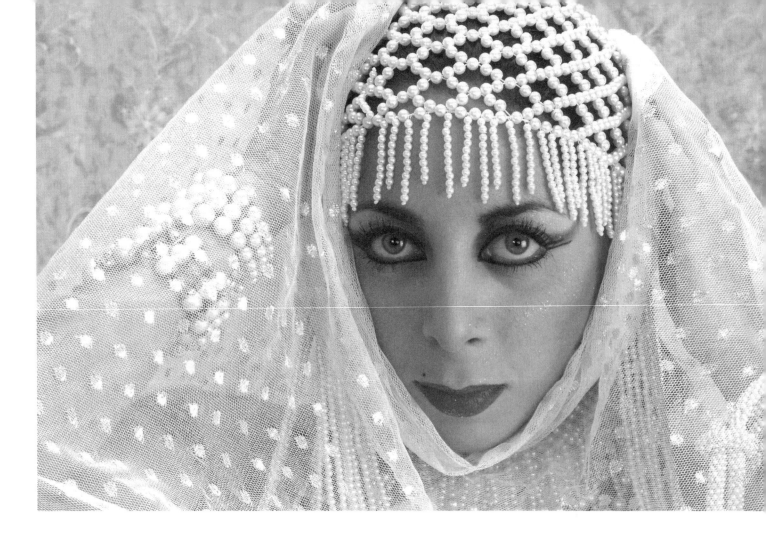

# Veils

A veil is the one essential part of a belly dancer's perform-ance costume that is also used in practice sessions. Veils are always associated with the Middle East. One thinks of veiled women, swirling veils, or Salome's Dance of the Seven Veils.

Actually, in the Middle East, a veil is a modesty garment, worn to shield women from the eyes of strangers. Traditionally, veils were never used as props for dance until the 20th century, when Egyptian dancer Samia Gamal appeared on stage with a large piece of fabric. She was taking lessons from a famous Russian ballerina who suggested that she use this piece of fabric to help her hold her arms better. The look caught on, and it soon became standard for dancers to make their entrances holding fabric "veils."

Forty years before Samia Gamal's veil debut, veils had already become associated with Middle Eastern dance in Western cultures because of Salome, the biblical temptress who demanded the head of John the Baptist on a platter as payment for dancing at King Herod's birthday party. But if you look in the bible, you'll find no mention of Salome using veils. (In fact, the bible doesn't even mention Salome by name; the dancer is referred to only as "the daughter of Herodias.") The Dance of the Seven Veils was created for the 1905 opera *Salome* by German composer Richard Strauss, based on Oscar Wilde's controversial play *Salome: A Tragedy in One Act*, which was considered so racy that it was banned in England and never performed on stage during Wilde's lifetime. Because of the play and the opera, the Western world became intrigued by the fantasy of Salome seductively removing seven veils one at a time. Although the Dance of the Seven Veils had absolutely nothing to do with genuine Middle Eastern dance, it soon became synonymous with the belly dancer's art.

Today, in Egypt and other Middle Eastern countries, a dancer glides onstage with a veil, uses it only for the first few minutes of her show, then discards it. In the United States, though, it became popular for belly dancers to use veils for slow songs, using them to create shapes and illusions. Some say the technique was imported by Turkish dancers in the 1960s. Now, belly dancers throughout the world use veils, both for fast, gliding entrances and with slow music.

## Shopping for a Veil

Vendors of belly dance supplies sell a variety of veils. I recommend those made of China silk. Many are artfully hand-dyed, sometimes combining several colors in beautiful designs.

Most of the veils that come from Egypt and Turkey are polyester. They usually have bead and sequin work around all the edges, which makes them heavier and more cumbersome than plain veils. That's because, in the Middle East, dancers use the veils only for simple entrances, so they like the showy sparkle, but they don't need the veils to flow. If you hit someone accidentally while dancing with a beaded veil, it might hurt. Needless to say, I don't recommend them. If I were buying a costume and the seller threw in an Egyptian or Turkish veil for free, I'd take it, but if you start out using one of them, you will

not fall in love with the sensuality of veil dancing—and you really should.

In this book, I'll only show how to use the basic rectangular veil, which is the most versatile and easiest to use. There are also other shapes, such as half-circles and fully circular capes. "Wings"—full-length capes made of pleated lamé or crystal organza—are growing in popularity in dance performances. They are quite dramatic, so you have lots to look forward to as you progress in your belly dance skills.

## Making Your Own Veil

The veil is simply a rectangular piece of lightweight fabric. The best size is three yards long by 45 inches wide.

The fabric should be very soft and translucent. The best fabric to buy is silk chiffon or smooth China silk. You can also use polyester chiffon, which comes in a wide variety of colors, is easier to find in fabric stores, and is quite reasonably priced. I prefer silk because it flows beautifully and feels so soft and sensual.

Before using the veil, you will need to finish the ends where the fabric has been cut. The long edges are already finished. You can either use a sewing machine set on the zigzag or hemming stitch, or hem it by hand. Silk must be sewn, but with polyester, you can save time by singeing the edge instead. To do this, run the cut end of the veil quickly through the outer vapors of a lit candle flame. Make sure your hair is tied back, and be careful not to put the fabric too close to the flame or hold it there too long. Singeing the edge is tricky at first, but quick once you get the hang of it.

If you want to add sparkle or shine to your veil, I suggest sewing paillettes (small, shiny, lightweight discs like sequins that you sew on) to the hemmed ends of the veil, but forget about using glass beads.

# Finger Cymbals

*F*inger cymbals (called *zils* in Turkish or *zagat* in Arabic) are an important part of Middle Eastern dance, adding life to your performance. It's not necessary to use them in your fitness workout—in fact, when starting out on your own, they can be one too many things to think about. In my opinion, playing finger cymbals while dancing is the hardest part of belly dancing. But if you're using this workout book for practice sessions between classes, of course you'll want to practice finger cym-

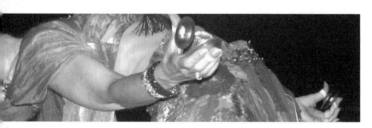

bals, too. As you progress, they will help you develop better coordination and become one with the music.

In the beginning, you might want to practice with finger cymbals while you're walking, not dancing. Playing along with your workout CD will help you get attuned to the often intricate rhythms of Middle Eastern music.

Finger cymbals, like other belly dance accessories, are available from many different sources—in dance studios and shops, at belly dance conventions, in mail-order catalogs, and on the Internet. Most dancers prefer to shop for them someplace where they can try before they buy, instead of sending away for them, because different cymbals have different sounds. They also come in different sizes, the larger ones being louder. For a

beginner, smaller ones—two inches in diameter—are better because they are lighter and somewhat easier to use. A dancer who performs where there is a lot of ambient noise, like in restaurants or a clubs, may prefer larger, louder ones.

The cymbals are attached to your fingers with elastic loops. Be sure to get ones with two parallel slots for the elastic; some cheaper ones have a single hole in the center, but they are harder to control. For the same reason, flat strips of elastic ("braid elastic") are better than round ones.

Before playing the finger cymbals, adjust the elastic so that they fit snugly and don't slip around on your finger. When you've adjusted them to the right size, either sew the elastic or secure them with a small safety pin. You may wish to use a safety pin for a while, since some elastic stretches out with use.

## Playing Finger Cymbals

Finger cymbals are the belly dancer's personal percussion instrument, and it's a good idea to start practicing with them at your first opportunity. The best way to understand Middle Eastern rhythms is to play along with them.

It takes a certain touch to make finger cymbals ring out instead of just clanking together. Place the cymbals securely on the thumb and middle finger of each hand. Listen to the music and figure out the downbeat by stepping or clapping your hands in time to the music. That beat is "single time." Double, triple, and quadruple time are simply multiplications of the single downbeat. You'll normally strike the cymbals on one hand, then the other, not both at the same time. Practice these, always starting with your right hand (unless you are left-handed):

| | 1 | 2 | 3 | 4 |
|---|---|---|---|---|
| *Single time* | R | L | R | L |
| *Double time* | RL | RL | RL | RL |
| *Triple time* | RLR | RLR | RLR | RLR |
| *Quadruple time* | RLRL | RLRL | RLRL | RLRL |

Once you've gotten the hang of these simple rhythms, start working on the most important rhythms used in belly dance, the *malfuf* and the *beledi*.

| | 1 | 2 | 1 | 2 |
|---|---|---|---|---|
| *Malfuf* | R | RLRL | R | RLRL |
| *Malfuf variation* | clap | RLRL | clap | RLRL |

| | 1 | 2 | 3 | 4 | |
|---|---|---|---|---|---|
| *Beledi* | RR | RLR | R | RLR | |
| *Beledi w/Bridge** | RR | RLR | R | RLR | (RL) |
| *Beledi variation* | clapclap | RLR | clap | RLR | |

\* the bridge is a quick RL on the upbeat

There are many other rhythms in Middle Eastern dance; as you progress, you'll pick them up through classes or listening to music.

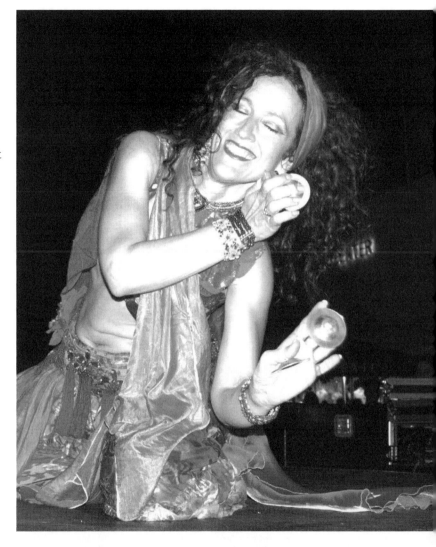

# Music

the subject of Middle Eastern music is vast, as you will discover if you get deeply involved in belly dance. In fact, it will add a whole new dimension to your CD collection. For now, I will try not to bore you, and make it as straightforward as possible.

There are many styles of music to choose from. We can begin by putting them into three basic categories, though they could be broken down into dozens, and if you include the various ethnic styles, they would become even more numerous. Let's start with just these three: (1) Pop, (2) Oriental, and (3) Traditional.

Pop music became a belly dance staple around 1990. It was a big change from Oriental and traditional styles, and dancers took to it immediately.

Middle Eastern pop music usually comes from Egypt, Lebanon, or Turkey. The Egyptian pop style is the one most commonly used for belly dancing, combining traditional folk and belly dance rhythms with a contemporary driving sound augmented by synthesizers. Of the many famous Egyptian pop singers, the ones most known outside the Middle East are Hakim and Amr Diab. Of course, just as in American pop music, hot new singing stars explode onto the scene weekly.

From Lebanon, big names include Ragheb Alama and Diana Haddad. Turkey rocketed into the world music scene with "The Kiss Song" by Tarkan.

Algerian *rai*, a kind of music that originally focused on social commentary, is now mainstream in dance clubs throughout the world. There are many famous names, starting with Cheb Khaled and Cheb Mami ("Cheb" means young). Rai is occasionally, though not often, used in belly dance performances, but it's good music for warm-ups.

When dancers put together a belly dance tape or CD for a performance, they usually try to avoid relying too much on pop. It can dilute the dance if the structure of a show or routine is allowed to deteriorate from the complexities of Oriental compositions and the sensitivity of traditional acoustic music to one pop song after another. Like disco, a whole playlist of Middle Eastern pop music can result in a continuum of steady rhythm with no beginning, middle, or end. On the other hand, pop music is great in a nightclub setting, where the audience can relate to the even and contagious beats and feel encouraged to dance along with the dancer.

Oriental music, as the term is used in belly dance, doesn't mean Chinese or Japanese. It means "Eastern," including Middle Eastern, as opposed to "Western" music; it's a translation from the Arabic word *sharqi*. Oriental music came into its golden age from the 1930s on, when it was elaborated for lavish nightclub floor shows and movies with musical dance numbers. Great composers that came out of that era include Mohamed Abdel Wahab and Farid El Atrache, among many others. They either composed songs for a particular movie or were commissioned to create music for a dancer or singer. They used a variety of rhythms and arranged their songs for large orchestras of musicians, the main instruments being violins, percussion, oud, khanoun, and accordion. Many songs of that era are still used in belly dance today, in both original and updated versions.

New Oriental music is constantly composed at the request of present-day dancers. Nagwa Fouad, an Egyptian dancer whose fame reached its peak in the 1980s, commissioned some of the most popular pieces we dance to. Among them are "Mashaal," "Banat Eskanderia," and "Set El Hosen." Other popular Oriental pieces for dancing were originally composed as preludes for songs for famous singers. "Batswanis Beek" and "Fi Youm Wi Leila" were written for the singer Warda. "1001 Nights," "Leilat Hob," and "Inta Omri" are just a few from the top Egyptian singer of all time, the legendary Oum Khalthoum.

*Aziza* is to an Arabic band playing for belly dancers as "New York, New York" would be for an American wedding band; in other words, everyone knows it. Professional belly dancers know that the above listed songs are safe bets to ask any Arabic band to play for their performances.

Traditional music was played by entirely acoustic musicians or groups. When I started dancing, acoustic music was the most popular for belly dancing, but it's not so common now. A traditional belly dance show would be a series of fast songs strung together by *taksims*, arrhythmic improvisations played with a single instrument. The show would end with a drum solo and fast finale.

For performances, belly dancers usually prefer a structured six-part show, paced to hold the audience's attention:

1. Fast opening
2. Slow song
3. Medium-tempo song with a steady beat
4. Slow song
5. Drum solo
6. Finale

The styles of music may vary, with an Oriental piece for the opening, a slow song second, a modern pop song third, a beautiful *taksim* fourth, and a peppy drum solo to give a high point to the show, then a one- to two-minute finale, which may be the end of the Oriental opening song.

# Middle Eastern Musical Instruments

Get to know about the instruments used in Middle Eastern music and listen for them. Even modern synthesized music involves these instruments because they are sampled into the synthesizer keyboard. Sometimes one keyboardist will be playing the sounds of several instruments, which has put a lot of tradi-

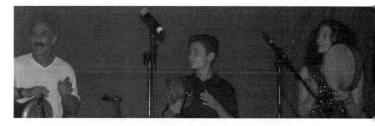

tional musicians out of business. A one- to three-man band can sound like an entire orchestra and save the nightclub owner a lot of money.

Of course, there is nothing like the real thing, and when synthesizers are used, acoustic instruments tend to get drowned out by overzealous keyboard players. The oud and khanoun are delicate and sensitive, and though they are the most traditional and beautiful, they are often ignored or left out altogether these days.

The most common Middle Eastern musical instruments are:

**Dumbek** (otherwise known as *tabla* or *darbuka*): The beat of the music is most important to dance to, and the dumbek keeps the beat. This hourglass-shaped drum is the rhythmic backbone for every style of Middle Eastern music, whether pop, Oriental, or traditional. Dumbeks were originally made of ceramic with fish skin or goat skin head, but now most are cast metal with plastic heads.

**Riqq**: This tambourine-like percussion instrument is used to keep a steady beat. The cymbals along the edges of the riqq are played with the fingers as well as the drum head.

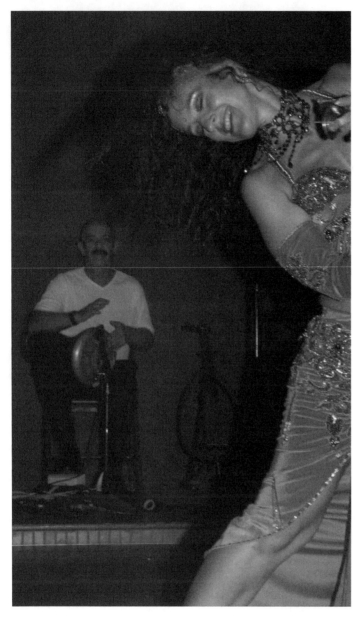

**Oud**: An egg-shaped stringed instrument with a big belly, this ancient precursor to the guitar is similar to the lute played in medieval European music.

**Khanoun**: This harplike stringed instrument lays flat and is played with metal tips worn over the fingers. It is quite intricate to play. The dancer can combine shimmies layered onto slow music to take advantage of the khanoun's full range of sounds.

**Kemanja**: This folk instrument, played upright with a bow, evolved into the violin in Europe. Today, violins have replaced the kemanja in all but the most folkloric Middle Eastern music. Sometimes an Oriental band will have several violinists.

**Accordion**: Based on one of the first Chinese musical instruments, European accordions were first made in Austria around 1830. Within a few years, they were introduced to Egyptian music and converted to accommodate the quarter tones in the Arabic musical scale. The accordion is a staple in Middle Eastern bands, and accordion *taksims* are wonderfully hypnotic. In a type of improvised song called the "beledi buildup," the accordion starts slow and gradually builds up into a series of accents, finally getting very fast as lots of drums join in.

**Clarinet**: Invented in Europe and first used in compositions by Handel and Mozart, the clarinet is a staple of Turkish music but not Arabic. Turkish clarinets are made of metal. In addition to playing *taksims*, they can get really fast and exciting.

## Rhythms

There are many rhythms in belly dance music. For anyone who is serious about belly dancing, it's a good idea to purchase a CD that focuses on and explains these rhythms. (A good one is Jalilah's *Raqs Sharqi 4* or Hossam Ramzy's *Rhythms of the Nile*.) Listen for the "downbeat"—the beat you clap to. That is the beat on which your weight should be down into the ground. For example, if you step, you step down on the downbeat. If you drop your hip, it goes down on the downbeat. Dropping the chest is also down on the downbeat.

**Mazhar**: This much bigger version of the tambourine has several layers of cymbals. It is heavy and requires considerable strength to play. In fact, some musicians say it's the hardest Middle Eastern instrument to play.

**Zaghat** (in Arabic, or *zils* in Turkish): Finger cymbals are typically used by belly dancers, but they are also played by musicians in bands. Sometimes musicians use a bigger version, which fits a man's hands and would be too cumbersome to dance with, but the sound really carries.

Here are some of the major rhythms, though there are many more. Some musicians disagree on the names or even how some rhythms are played, but the following are standard. When first learning to recognize them, you might want to drum on a table top or your knees with the palms of your hands to catch onto the rhythms. After you can identify the various rhythms on CDs, try playing along with finger cymbals.

## Rhythm Family #1:

**Beledi** (4/4), otherwise known as the "small masmoudi," goes Dum Dum Tek-i Tek, Dum Tek-i Tek. (On a dumbek, the *Dum* is played with the right hand near the center of the drum head, giving the beat a deep sound. The Tek is also played with the right hand, but on the edge of the drum head to sound crisp and light. The *i* is played on the edge, too, but with the left hand.)

**Maksum** (2/4) is like the beledi, but shorter: Dum Tek Tek, Dum Tek.

**Big masmoudi** (eight beats to the bar) is like the beledi but uses more beats: Dum Dum Tek-i-tek i-tek, Dum Tek-i-tek i-tek-i-tek-i-tek i.

## Rhythm Family #2

**Malfuf** (2/4), which means "rolling," is in two beats and goes 1-1234. You can remember it by saying the words "Shave and a haircut." It is played differently on the drum than it sounds when we play the finger cymbals.

**Ayub** (2/4) is a rhythm used for the "Zar," an ancient trance dance from Egypt. Its rhythm has made its way into belly dancing music, so a dancer should be aware of it and do a little bit of movement with the head to show acknowledgement of its roots. It is strong and earthy: Dum tek Dum Tek.

## Assorted Rhythms:

**Saidi** (4/4), from El Said in southern Egypt, is often used for cane dances, accompanied by a wind instrument called the mizmar. It is very similar to the beledi and can be played two ways: with one Dum then 2 (Dum Dum-dum), or using two and two (Dum-dum Dum-dum).

**Semai** (10/8) is a classical rhythm that occurs in both Turkish and Arabic music and dates back to the time when Arabs ruled Spain. It is in ten beats, and even the best musicians have a hard time agreeing on how it is played, but the accents are most important: Dum Dum Dum-Dum-Dum, or 1-2-123-hold hold. When dancing to a semai, it is important to be aware that this rhythm has pauses so wait for it to start again. The hardest thing to do in belly dancing is to hold still and not move, but that is part of the art and sensitivity to the music.

**Chifti telli** is a Turkish word, but the rhythm is also used in Arabic music. It is often played slow, though in Turkish and Greek styles it has fast versions as well. The Greeks call home-style belly dancing "Chifti Telli." It is in eight beats and goes: 1-2345-123.

The **Karshlima** or **Turkish 9/8** also comes in many varieties and is common in Turkish music. It was taken by the Gypsies (Roma) from Turkish folk music and adapted to the belly dance. It can be heard everywhere in Turkey, but never in the Arab world. It has nine beats and, simplified, can be interpreted as 1-2-3-123.

## Middle Eastern Music CDs

Whether you're taking classes or only working out on your own, you'll certainly want to buy at least one CD of Middle Eastern music to dance to. Ideally, you will begin to build a collection and select tracks to make your first belly dance CD or tape, as discussed in "Make Your Own Music" below.

There are thousands of great belly dance CDs to choose from. You can find some of them in the world music sections of stores that sell CDs. Wide assortments of Middle Eastern CDs are also sold by vendors at belly dance conventions, and at

Middle Eastern shops and belly dance supply stores in most large cities.

Look up "Middle Eastern music" on Internet search engines or browse through some of the websites listed in the "Resources" section of this book. Several websites that sell Middle Eastern CDs let you preview songs before you order. There are even some websites and online music services that let you buy songs one at a time in mp3 and mp4 format, which is great for burning your own workout or performance CD because you can buy only the songs you want from various CDs, and your own customized CD ends up costing you no more than a single commercial CD would.

*The following are excellent CDs to start your collection with:*

Jalilah, a Canadian dancer, has commissioned music in Egypt and Lebanon that encompasses a wide variety of Oriental styles, ranging from those composed in the golden age for films to songs created for famous Middle Eastern singers. Jalilah has released a series of six CDs titled *Jalilah's Raqs Sharqi*, and I recommend all of them. Number Four features all the rhythms and uses excerpts from songs on her other CDs to demonstrate how they sound when played with only drums and then when played with an orchestra—a valuable tool to help you understand the rhythms of Middle Eastern music.

Hossam Ramzy, a famous Egyptian percussionist as well as belly dance teacher, has dozens of CDs on the market. I most recommend *Rhythms of the Nile, Best of Oum Kolthoum, Best of Farid Al Atrache, Best of Mohammed Abdul Wahab*, and *Best of Abdul Halim Hafiz*. If your local music store doesn't have them, you can order them via the Internet from his website, www.hossamramzy.com.

For excellent compilations of the modern pop style, check out the two *Bellydance Superstars* CDs from Ark 21 Records. They feature music hand-picked by top dancers and teachers from around the United States. (The first volume features two tracks selected by me.)

You'll find more discussion of Middle Eastern music in "Belly Dance Lore" later in this part of the book.

## Make Your Own Music

I use a sound system with a CD burner to create my own music CDs for classes and performances, and it's a good idea to do the same for your own workouts at home. If your sound system is an older model, you can record songs from commercial CDs onto a cassette tape. However, it's best to use a 120-minute cassette, recording a full hour-long practice set on each side, so you don't have to stop midway through your workout to turn the tape over. Your CD or tape should follow this sequence:

- Five or six slow songs—try New Age music by Vas, the *Scheherazade Suite*, or slow pieces from your favorite Middle Eastern CDs.
- Two drum solos—good ones can be found on *Bellydance Superstars*, volume 1 or 2, or Jalilah's *Raqs Sharqi*, volume 1, 2, 3, 5, or 6.
- Four medium-tempo songs with a steady beat—there are several of these songs on both *Bellydance Superstars*, both volumes 1 and 2.
- One or two songs with varied beats—try two from *Bellydance Superstars*, Volume 1 track 1, 4, or 5, or one of the longer ones from Jalilah's *Raqs Sharqi*, Volume 1 track 1, Volume 2 track 2, Volume 3 track 1 or 2, or Volume 6 track 1.
- One nice cool-down song—you will love the title track of Cirque du Soleil's *Egypte*.

Once you have compiled this CD or tape, you can use it every time you practice from start to finish, going through all the movements (depending on how many weeks you have been practicing). When you crave a change of music, just make another CD with the same format.

# costumes

You don't need a costume to belly dance in, but you may want one for fun. It is important to dress appropriately for your age, body type, and the music you are using. Unlike ballet or jazz, which are youth-oriented, belly dance only ripens and improves with age. A woman can continue dancing all her life and only become more beautiful and proficient.

There are many options. You can spend $400 to $1000 on the high-end costumes imported from Egypt or Turkey, elaborate, hand-beaded, and often adorned with crystals. Or you can get creative and make your own. When I started, all dancers had to make their own costumes. Each of my early costumes took between one to six months to bead by hand. Now, you can save time by cutting up old beaded dresses from thrift shops and using ready-made trims.

Another costume option is the "beledi dress," which is a one-piece caftan that is worn for cane dances and other earthier dance styles. These can be embellished with hipscarves, headpieces, and coined jewelry. A caftan can also be a great addition to the belly dance enthusiast's wardrobe. You can use it to cover a costume on the way to a performance, wear it as a costume with a sash tied at the hips, or get in the Middle Eastern spirit and wear it as an evening dress when attending a belly dance show, gala, or Middle Eastern–themed dinner party.

If you are going to perform, even if it is a simple setting like a friend's party or retirement home, getting ready is half the fun. Make sure your hair and makeup look good. You can wear a hairpiece or leave your hair natural, but make sure it is neat and has some style. Make sure the back of your bra is secured by extra safety pins, that it fits properly, and that you have prac-

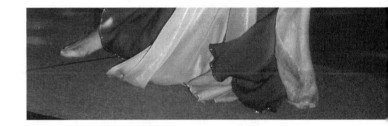

*Good taste is of utmost importance in costuming and what is concealed is more important than what is revealed.*

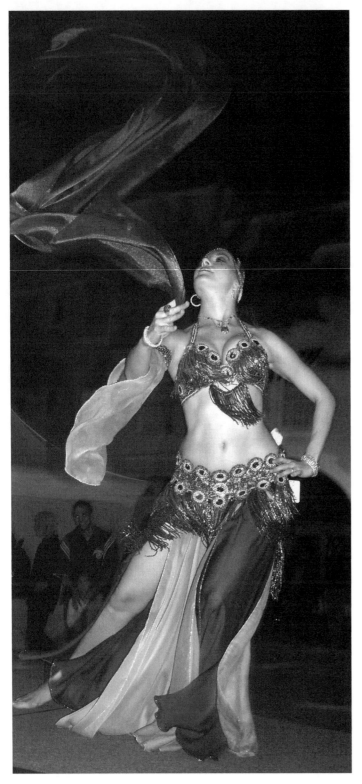

ticed dancing with it at home to make sure it doesn't ride up or gap. If you are wearing a hip scarf or belt that is separate from the costume, make sure it is pinned securely. I encourage dancers to wear matching shorts under their costumes, especially when dancing on a raised stage.

Some dancers wear shoes, while others prefer going barefoot. The choice is yours, but if the surface you dance on is rough, you may want to protect your feet. For a fancy costume, you can wear gold or silver ballroom dance shoes. More casual looks can go with lace-up Hermes sandals or suede dance thongs that cover only the front of the foot (both available at dance stores). Both types of costuming look good with gold or silver flat slippers, which are popular among Egyptian dancers.

Always accessorize. Use headbands, turbans, flowers in the hair, big, shiny earrings, necklaces, bracelets, etc. Carry that exotic look from head to toe.

# PART 2

# The World of Belly Dancing

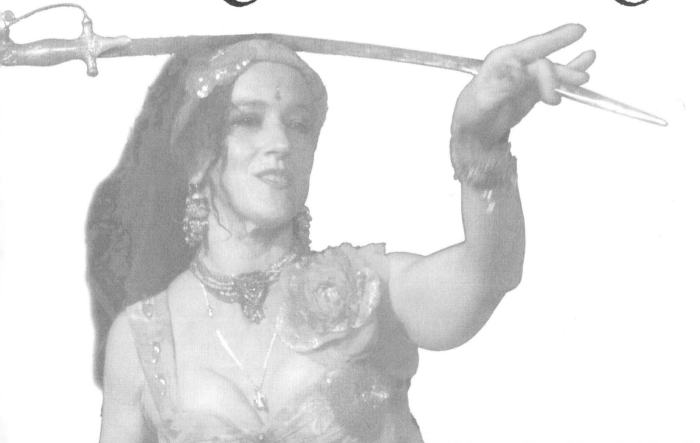

# History

Dance historians believe that belly dance began as a childbirth ritual in ancient times. There were no hospitals, and no pain killers or other pharmaceuticals were available to women giving birth, so natural childbirth was the only option available. It makes sense that women would ritualize movements that strengthened and toned the muscles that would make childbirth easier.

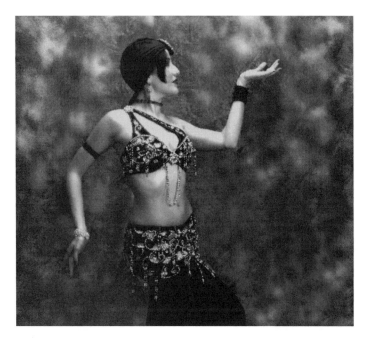

You'll notice that many belly dance movements are centered in the pelvic or abdominal area. A combination of muscle control and relaxation, they exercise the internal organs and tone the stomach muscles and waistline. Undulating movements actually use muscles that push the baby out of the womb.

Some people theorize that these movements may have been set to music and ritualized as part of a women's "goddess" religion that spread throughout the ancient Middle Eastern world. Though it is widely believed that ancient feminine religions were suppressed by the rise of patriarchal religions,

including Judaism, Christianity, and Islam, it may well be that echoes of primeval goddess worship ceremonies live on in the art of belly dance today, though very far removed.

The term "belly dance" comes from the Arabic word *beledi*, meaning "of the people." Beledi is used to refer to music, dance, and costuming. It has nothing to do with anatomy. Since its origins, beledi has always been a dance of feminine expression, performed most often among women and out of the sight of men.

Beledi evolved into a multicultural art form known today as "Oriental dance" during the Ottoman Empire, when women from many countries lived together in the harems of Turkish sultans. The women of the harems had plenty of time on their hands, and you can bet they danced! Of course, many lucky sultans were entertained by dancers, but the women often were only seen as shadows undulating behind a latticework screen. The eroticism of belly dance comes from the mystery of the forbidden and unseen.

Men have been fascinated by the "belly dance" not only because of its innate and uninhibited sensuality but also because of the mystery of not being allowed into women's quarters and women-only celebrations of which the dance was—and still is—an integral part. European Orientalist painters saw, or at least heard about, prostitutes who were the only women available to Western eyes. This led them to fantasize about the Middle Eastern women they could not see. They passionately painted harem scenes from their imaginations, even though some of these painters never left Europe but merely imagined through their art.

In 1893, Oscar Wilde's play *Salome* was banned in England for its "lewd" dance. Also in 1893, American promoter Sol Bloom brought a troupe of real North African folk dancers to the Chicago World's Fair and coined the term "belly dance."

Belly dancers (often imitators with no knowledge of Middle Eastern culture), or "exotic dancers," as they were often known, become a central part of vaudeville and burlesque stage shows, and this dance form soon abandoned its Middle Eastern roots to become confused with striptease. Long after vaudeville had become outmoded and faded away, belly dance retained a slightly naughty reputation.

When I got my start as a professional dancer, it was in vogue to send "bellygrams" to people on their birthdays, which offered young dancers a way to earn money and gain performing experience without compromising their dignity. Most women who get into belly dance as merely a way to make money eventually realize the difficulty, skill, and practice required to reach a professional level and give it up for a faster, easier way to make a buck. It's not about shaking our bodies to excite men! Belly dance can be made commercial and silly, but it would never have survived for so many millennia if it were so superficial.

Today, women around the world have reclaimed belly dance and transformed it into something much closer to its original roots. Some study for exercise, while others love the music or the mystique of Middle Eastern culture. The vast majority of women who develop a passion for belly dance as an art form get hooked on the mystery that unfolds as one complex layer of isolations leads to more ways to use our bodies, expressing everything from gutsy, matriarchal feminine power to ethereal spiritual expression. When they least expect it, the dance transports them to another aspect of their being that has yet to be discovered.

This dance is about mystery—the mystery of ancient culture, foreign to most of us, deep and complex. The mystery of muscle control; the mystery of our own bodies. The mystery of music that has different rhythms, instruments, and tones than Western music. The mysterious moments when you are one with the music. The mystery of your energy, and of how the melding of energies becomes magic.

# Egyptian, Turkish, & Lebanese Belly Dancing Styles

"Belly dance" is a catch-all term that does not exist in the Middle East. It can mean raks beledi, which is done in a long dress with a scarf tied at the hip. Or it can mean Oriental dance, which is a fusion of Egyptian-style beledi with Persian, Turkish, and even Indian influences.

Some people feel that the only "real" belly dance is the Egyptian style. I don't agree. Yes, the great and beloved dancers of the silver screen were Egyptian. Samia Gamal, Naima Akef, and Tahia Carioca were household names throughout the Arab world because when black-and-white musicals were the rage in Hollywood, filmmakers in Cairo started their own film industry, and it took the Middle East by sandstorm. Long ago, belly dancers didn't wear fancy costumes. They just wore clothes like everyone else, but tied scarves around their hips. Inspired by Hollywood, the Egyptian film industry added sparkle (sequins), jingle (coins), and flesh (bare bellies and sheer skirts). They created elaborate tableaus with Busby Berkeleyesque choreographies. The previously popular folksy music developed into a "golden age," and composers such as smoldering actor-singer Farid El Atrache and Mohamed Abdel Wahab, who was the first to add some original Western touches, became superstars.

The next generation of belly dancers could be seen around the world in 1980s belly dance videos, Egypt's answer to MTV. Among them were Nagwa Fouad, Souhair Zaki, and Fifi Abdo. Nagwa staged big shows with lots of dancers and singers, and the music composed especially for her is still popular with performers today.

Souhair Zaki was the first belly dancer respected enough to dare dance to the music of Egyptian singer Oum Kulthoum, who was so revered that she was often referred to simply as "the lady," and whose songs lasted up to 90 minutes each. When her radio program aired, the Arab-Israeli war was put on hold until she finished singing before they resumed their fighting. After Souhair Zaki performed to Oum Kulthoum's overtures on videos, belly dancers around the world started to do the same. Now, long after Oum Kulthoum's death, there are funky disco-bellydance versions of her songs . . . .

The dancers of the silver screen have passed away, Nagwa and Souhair have retired, and Fifi is still on the scene. There is a new generation of dancers in Egypt, most notably Dina, who shocks the world with her daring costumes, which are illegal under Egyptian modesty laws, but she is so famous that she gets away with anything she wants.

Raqia Hassan is Egypt's leading and most active dance teacher. She organizes the yearly "Ahlan Wa Sahlan" Dance Festival of Cairo, which attracts belly dancers from around the world. She also travels to teach workshops in the United States, Europe, and Asia. When in Cairo, she teaches privately in her home and takes breaks to cook for her students and encourage them to "Eat . . . eat!" Raqia never performed belly dance in public but was a lead dancer in the Mahmoud Reda folkloric troupe, the first folk ballet that was respected enough in the Middle East to perform in theaters and films, starting in the 1950s. Troupe organizer Mahmoud Reda, who is now a gentle silver-haired man in his 80s, still tours and teaches dance workshops around the world.

Obviously, Egypt is a major player in the belly dance scene, so where do the Turks fit in? In Turkey, the Roma (Gypsies) had a major role in the development of belly dancing. The Roma originated in India and absorbed and adapted music and dance styles from every land they traveled to. Their genius musicians, who never followed the rules, permanently changed the sound of Turkish music, adapting classical Ottoman styles and traditional Turkish folk rhythms, while the women mixed belly dance with their own big skirts, hops, turns, and raw, earthy appeal—and out came the Turkish Roma style.

The Ottoman Empire lasted hundreds of years and spanned countries ranging from the Balkans of Eastern Europe to Yemen, Iraq, Syria, and parts of North Africa including Egypt. The performers who entertained Ottoman sultans and their courts were commonly Jews, Roma musicians, and Turkish dancing boys who dressed as women. The Roma spread their style of music and belly dance movements to Bulgaria, Greece, the former Yugoslavia, and even into Romania. The best finger cymbal players are Turkish. Most people regard me as a good finger cymbal player, but when I spent time among the Roma in Turkey, I felt like a beginner.

In the 1990s, "Arabesque" songs—modern Egyptian pop songs sung in Arabic with a driving beat and modern instrumentation—became the rage in Turkey. Almost all belly dancers started performing to the upbeat Arabesque music, and it was played everywhere—on buses, in restaurants and shops, and so on. The biggest hits for belly dancing were a series of CDs called *mezdeke*, compilations of Egyptian pop songs. Finally, the Turkish government clamped down and decreed that, because traditional Turkish culture was being lost, belly dancers could not dance to music with Arabic words. A lot of bands started playing their own musical compositions with an Arabic style—but no words. The Turkish musicians have a knack for putting their own twist onto Arabic music and making it fun, unpredictable, and bursting with Turkish spirit.

The famed Colombian pop singer Shakira, who incorporates belly dance moves into her Latin rock, enjoys popularity that has swept the world. A lot of young girls have taken to imitating her style, as I saw when I visited Turkish Roma families in 2002. Their mothers weren't happy about their daughters dancing Shakira style instead of their own.

Lebanon, too, has made many contributions to belly dance. The famed dancer Nadia Gamal was very popular in the 1960s and '70s. She had a fast and feminine style all her own. Lebanon, a place of style, posh nightlife, and great cuisine, lent itself to the popularization of belly dancing. Unfortunately, civil war broke out, and arts slowed to a standstill. In the last ten years there has been a resurgence in Lebanon's music and dance industry.

Dancers there are thinner, appealing more to Western ideals of beauty. They wear high-heeled shoes and incorporate a smattering of jazz steps and inventive, homespun belly dance along with Egyptian, Turkish, and American influences.

## New Age & American Tribal Belly Dancing Styles

Belly dance is contagious, and it's spreading fast. Women around the world relate to it, and over many years it has metamorphosed into new forms. One of them, part of the New Age movement, is often called Goddess dancing. The slow movements and veils of belly dancing lend themselves well to meditative New Age music, and many American women have made a career of promoting this style of dance.

Another distinctly American style is called American Tribal. It emphasizes the exotic, much as did the Orientalist paintings of the 1800s, which were often created by artists who had never set foot in the Middle East. American Tribal was started in San Francisco in the 1960s by the American dancer Jamila Salimpour. Jamila, who pioneered belly dance on the U.S. West Coast, was dedicated to researching Middle Eastern and North African dances, music, and costuming. She wrote several books and articles, codified and named many of the steps with names that are still used today, started a school, owned a night club, and formed a dance troupe called Bal Anat.

When I started belly dancing in Seattle in 1976, the major influence was Jamila's tribal style. You might think that this style comes from some sort of authentic tribe, but it is actually a new hybrid "tribe," born in the U.S. Jamila fused dances and costuming from many different Middle Eastern and North African countries, and from different periods in history. For example, you might see one American Tribal dancer wearing the clothing of the Ottoman period in Egypt: a coat worn over a coined bodice and harem pants, combined with Afghan jewelry and Algerian facial tattoos painted on with eyeliner. Another

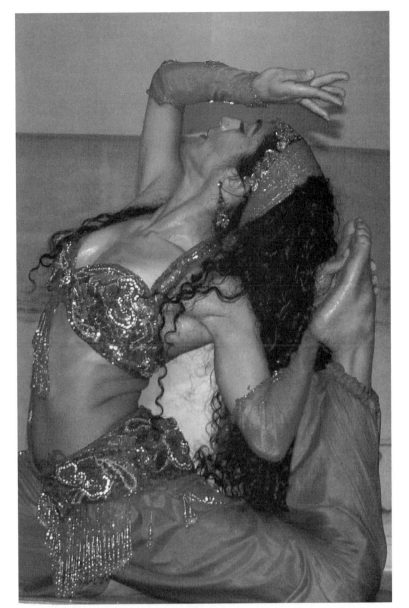

might wear a Tunisian costume instead, but her repertoire might consist of a mixture of belly dance and folklore from Turkey, Tunisia, Lebanon, and Egypt.

Jamila also created the sword dance from a European painting of an Egyptian dancer in the 1800s dancing for soldiers with one of their swords balanced on her head. Today, sword dancing is a normal part of the belly dance in the United States, Asia, Australia, Europe, and South America, and has progressed far beyond its American Tribal origins. I dance regularly with one or more swords for Middle Eastern audiences who know that it is not done in their countries, but love it just the same.

In the early '90s, a Brazilian belly dancer, Giselle Bomentre, was headed to Lebanon to try her luck. She wrote to ask my permission to dance with the sword in Lebanon, thinking that I had invented the sword dance since I was the first person she had seen use it in Brazil back in the 1980s. I explained that it is common in the United States and that I have no claim to it. Giselle became a star in the Middle East and stayed for ten years, appearing on television and in hotels throughout the Arabian Gulf, developing her own distinctive style, far different from the American Tribal style where sword dancing had started. Her costumes were made in Lebanon, with full chiffon skirts, elaborately beaded bras and belts, and high-heeled shoes, and she used the sword incorporating splits and ballet moves.

American Tribal continued as the main style on the West Coast until the dance community had more contact with the Egyptian style thanks to belly dance videos. Many dancers were bewitched by this new look and the refined techniques of Souhair Zaki and Nagwa Fouad, and their styles changed. By the end 1980s, the American Tribal style was seen mainly in the San Francisco area. Jamila Salimpour passed on her role as teacher to her 14-year-old daughter Suhaila, who remains one of the country's prominent belly dance teachers to this day. Suhaila traveled to Egypt and Lebanon, learning and performing, and studied all the Western styles of dance as well, including modern and jazz. Taking a different direction from her mother, she explored the many new options that opened to her. Years later, the American Tribal style enjoyed a resurgence, and today it is growing in popularity by leaps. Recently, Jamila Salimpourhas began teaching again.

A Bay Area dancer named Carolena Nericcio created a troupe called Fat Chance Belly Dance, which had a feminist slant, wore black Indian Gypsy skirts, cholis (Indian crop tops), big turbans with roses, and Afghan jewelry, and sported genuine tattoos on their stomachs. They used music with a heavily ethnic sound, such as Nubian, Saudi, or other folk sounds, and combined Middle Eastern and Flamenco postures with lots of belly rolls, stomach flutters, finger cymbals, group dances, and serious, intense expressions.

Carolena's dances were so mystical and captivating that the troupe developed a wide following. With a a knack for promotion, she marketed instructional videos, music, sewing patterns, and a plethora of products to share her unique vision of American Tribal belly dance. Across the United States, in towns big and small, video viewers took the Fat Chance Belly Dance course and followed it step for step. A new generation of lookalike Fat Chance Belly Dance troupes sprang up like mushrooms in the most unlikely places, from Appalachia to Alaska.

Today there are American Tribal festivals, and the style has taken hold at renaissance festivals. Thanks to American Tribal's well developed network, new artists continue to come forth who love this style and make it their own, and it is developing respect as a major branch of belly dancing, as well as new, individual and artistic takes on this unique fusion.

## The Belly Dance Subculture

Belly dancing can be addictive. At some point, it becomes hard to go a day without undulating. You miss it . . . your muscles miss the movement. You know you're hooked when all the CDs in your car are belly dance music, and your voicemail message contains belly dance music. When you practice dancing, you reaffirm a connection with the entire little-known community of women around the world and across the centuries who share a passion for this dance.

Over the years, many of your friends will be the people you've met in belly dance class. That camaraderie extends to the network of women who meet up at belly dance classes, festivals, and conventions in their home towns and across the world.

# PART 3

# Your Workout Plan

# fundamentals

## The Importance of Posture

Imagine looking at a beautiful painting in a broken frame, or playing a bent saxophone. Belly dancing with bad posture is like that. You can do the greatest moves, but they just won't come out right unless you have the proper posture.

If I had to choose between seeing a person do dozens of fancy movements with poor posture or a few simple movements with beautiful posture, I would opt for simplicity.

Good posture makes it easier to do the belly dance movements. Belly dancing requires *isolation,* which means separating each part of your body. The only way to do that is to be relaxed and keep your spine elongated to the tallest possible position. That way, there is more room to move, and you are better positioned to do the movements.

Belly dancing can be excellent therapy for your back, but only if done with good posture. If you slouch or arch, you can actually pull muscles and feel pain in your back.

The optimal posture for belly dancing (or just about anything else, for that matter) is with your shoulders back, chest lifted and slightly forward. Keep your chin up, your stomach pulled in, and your hips tucked slightly under. One of the biggest benefits of belly dancing is the way your posture changes, which is good for you inside and out.

Try looking in the mirror as you practice standing in different postures: slouch, arch, and the belly dance posture. Notice how each one makes you look, then think about how each makes you feel.

Changing your posture is one of the most difficult things to do, but don't get discouraged. Once you become aware of how beneficial the change can be and how good you look and feel when you stand straight, you can practice it in your everyday life. The act of being consciously aware of your posture facilitates the change.

The way you hold yourself tells a lot about who you are and how you see or feel about yourself. Slouching can project an image of lack of energy or of low self-esteem. Using the belly dance posture in your everyday life gives you more energy and flexibility and projects an image of self-assurance. This posture also makes you look taller and gives your body a better proportion, making your clothes look better on you.

So go ahead. Lift your chest, pull your stomach in, and go out into the world with a new outlook. Soon it will become second nature. Don't wait until your dance workout or class to stand up straight.

## Relaxation Is the Key

When you think of femininity, what comes to mind? Most likely, softness is at the top of the list, but "soft" does not mean weak. Being soft, self-assured, and comfortable in your own skin and having fluid, graceful movements comes from one thing: relaxation.

The Western concept of "high-energy" often involves tension and strong, sharp movements. But that approach will not work with belly dancing, which comes from the Eastern school of thought. That means: stretch, release your tension, and go inside of the music instead of on top of it. In other words, the goal is to be part of the flow.

Until recently, belly dancers always performed with live musicians. Most Middle Eastern musicians use a lot of improvisation. Although they typically have a large repertoire of set songs, they never play the same song in the same way twice. Like jazz musicians, they jam, and to do that, they must be sensitive to one another and to the mood of the evening, and they must know how to flow. That takes relaxation. The dancer should be as one with the musicians, and that also requires relaxation.

Even though today we often use recorded music, belly dance is traditionally an improvised art form, and we must respond to the people and the space (or lack of) we have to dance in. We have to be dancing in the moment, and that too requires relaxation.

Relaxation is also therapeutic—a sort of meditation in motion. Modern life is stressful, and stress takes a toll on our bodies, causing any number of illnesses. Muscle tension causes everything from back and chest pains to problems with our shoulders, neck, and hands. Placing importance on relaxation as you practice belly dancing will make you feel so much better, and it helps avoid injuries as well.

The movements of belly dance call for a lot of strength and flexibility, but to make them look good, they must be done in a relaxed manner. You have to let the movement happen, not "make" it happen. One of the reasons that learning to belly dance takes time is that we have to switch from being hyper, tense Westerners to relaxing into the soft, fluid, and feminine movements that flow through Middle Eastern songs with age-old roots.

Don't expect to do it all overnight. Give the dance time to become natural for your body.

When you do a head slide, it will seem so difficult until you realize what is stopping you: tight muscles in the back of your neck. Once you let go of that tension, the head slide will seem

quite natural. The same principle applies to many movements, as you will see throughout the lessons in this book.

## Being Grounded

No, I don't mean "grounded" like when you did something bad as a teenager and had to stay home. Being grounded is a way of using your energy and your weight.

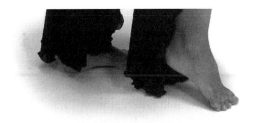

When you dance, keep in mind that in ancient times, women danced on the bare earth, maybe sand or maybe on hand-loomed rugs inside of tents. Their energy was very connected to the earth.

When you stand or do a dance step, take care to notice how your feet are placed. If one or both heels comes off the ground, it is for a reason, not by accident. Many movements require that both heels stay on the ground. If you lift your heel when you don't need to, the movement will not come out right.

Try standing with both feet flat on the floor. Feel the floor with your feet. Where is your weight—on the balls of your feet or on the heels?

Now, switch your weight from the balls of your feet to your heels and back again, without lifting your heels off the ground. Just become aware of your connection with the ground. Even if you are at the top of a highrise building, imagine the ground far below and extend the energy through your heels all the way to the earth below.

Without lifting either foot, switch your weight from one foot to the other and be aware of your body's relationship to the floor. That's what I mean by being grounded.

When you are grounded, your energy is focused. If you are not grounded, your energy can dissipate into the air, and then who knows where it goes? Certainly not into your dance.

Even if you are on your toes, you should feel the earth's gravity. If your upper body is lifted, or if you are looking up into the sky, you can be grounded from the waist down.

When you step, it is not necessary to step hard. You should always be graceful and not make noise with your feet. Just let go and sink a little bit with each step, as if you were dancing on warm sand.

Hip circles require that both feet stay flat on the floor. It is imperative that while doing the outside, horizontal figure-eight with your hips, you stay connected to the earth and use your knees to dip down. With the horizontal inside eight, you lift one heel and then the other, but you must make sure that both heels return to the floor, grounding you, before lifting the other heel.

When doing the V-step, you must always step flat when you cross, or else you will get stuck and find yourself unable to continue.

These are a few examples of the importance of grounding yourself. With all the movements I demonstrate in this book, notice where my feet are and how the weight is distributed.

Don't worry about analyzing what you have just read. Simply keep it in the back of your mind when you do the exercises in this book, and reread this advice after you have been practicing for several sessions.

## Lifting from the Chest

As the energy pulls you toward the earth from your feet and lower body, you must always remain as tall as possible and lift from your chest. This also uses ethereal energy, which is not in conflict with the earthiness I wrote about in the last section.

Imagine a string attached to the top of your head, pulling you up as high as you can go without leaving the ground. Your shoulders stay down, but your neck grows long. Pulling the shoulders gently back, the chest opens. This can be interpreted as opening your heart—letting the sun shine in.

Lift your chest, lengthening the waist as long as possible, and take a deep breath. With your chest up and forward, you should feel lighter and more free to do the hip movements that take place only from the waist down, as well as upper body isolations. Your arms will feel lighter and move with more grace and ease.

Lifting your chest makes you look taller and longer, and encourages you to pull in your stomach. Sometimes a dancer may be short in real life, but when she performs, everyone's perception is that she is very tall. This is because she lifts her chest.

Take a look in the mirror, standing normally. Then lift your chest and chin, and pull your shoulders back, stomach in. Notice how different you look.

Now, notice the difference in the way you feel.

Lastly, as you are lifting, don't forget to breathe. Take a few deep breaths and try to balance your earth energy with the ethereal energy. Feel the ground below your feet. Feel your spine expanding and your chest opening up. Use that feeling as a base from which to work as you learn to belly dance.

Some dancers are described as earthy, others as ethereal. Those qualities go with the personality, but with practice you can have it all—the best of both worlds.

# combinations & choreography

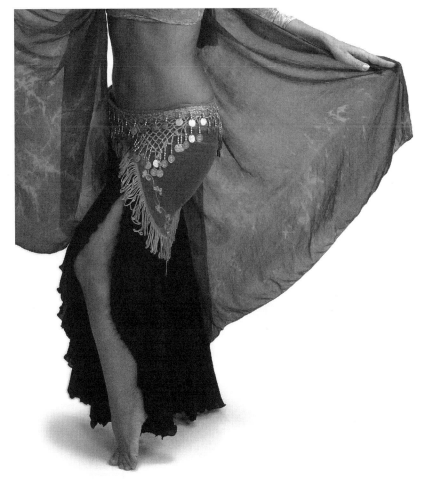

**B**elly dance is not a rigid art form based on choreography or limited technique. Once you know the basic movements, you constantly strive to improve your technique as a tool for expressing yourself, dancing out your own individuality. Choreography is used for performances, especially those by more than one dancer; although choreography is used extensively in Egypt and Lebanon, it is a nontraditional Western concept, added to belly dance during the 20th century.

Belly dance is typically improvised. In live performance, the musicians may take an established song and improvise within it, much like jazz. The dancer improvises, too. Sometimes the musicians follow her; other times she follows them. It is an exchange of energy.

A dance performance is like writing a story, with an opening, middle, and end. There is an established format for opening movements, using mellow walking, turning, or skipping steps with the veil. The middle can be whatever the dancer, musicians, and audience make it. The closing is, again, simple and unobtrusive, including walking, skipping, and turning.

As soon as you feel comfortable with the individual movements, try putting them together in the "Easy" combinations that follow in the chart on page 40. Repeat the same sequence of movements for the duration of the song. In the following weeks, as you learn more movements, move on to the "Medium" and "Challenging" ones. Once you learn how the movements flow into one another, unleash your imagination and invent your own combinations.

| | SLOW MUSIC | DRUM SOLO | MEDIUM-TEMPO MUSIC |
|---|---|---|---|
| **EASY COMBOS** | 1. Four-count Sunrise Arms two times.<br>2. Four Shoulder Circles: RLRL.<br>3. Four Ribcage Slides: RLRL.<br>4. Two two-count Medium Hip Circles to the right, two to the left. | 1. Four-count Hip Shimmy.<br>2. Four-count Hip Twist.<br>3. Four-count Shoulder Shimmy.<br>4. Four-count Hip Shimmy on toes. | 1. Four Egyptian Basics, starting right.<br>2. Four V-steps, starting with the left foot crossing front.<br>3. Four Scissor Steps with the left, then four with the right.<br>4. Four Shuffles to the left, then four to the right. |
| **MEDIUM COMBOS** | 1. Two two-count Ribcage Circles to the left, two to the right.<br>2. Four-count Sunrise Arms with four Hand Circles. Repeat four Hand Circles with Sunset Arms.<br>3. Cross your wrists at the level of your chest and do four Head Slides.<br>4. Two two-count Pelvic Undulations. | 1. Four Hip Drops with right, step flat, and Twist both hips, four counts.<br>2. Four Hip Twists with left on the ball of your left foot, step flat, and Hip Shimmy, four counts.<br>3. Four Hip Twists with right on the ball of your right foot.<br>4. Walk forward with four counts of Shoulder Shimmies. | 1. Four Hip Drops with a Kick with the right. Four Crescents with the right.<br>2. Four Hip Drops with a Kick with the left. Four Crescents with the left.<br>3. Four Suzy Qs: RLRL.<br>4. Walk forward: 1-2-3-clap. Then walk backward: 1-2-3-clap. |
| **CHALLENGING COMBOS** | 1. Four counts of Figure Eights horizontal inward: RLRL.<br>2. Four counts of Figure Eights horizontal outward: LRLR.<br>3. Four counts of Figure Eights vertical inward: RLRL.<br>4. Four counts of Figure Eights vertical outward: LRLR.<br>5. Four walks forward with Undulations (eight-count).<br>6. Four walks backward with Undulations (eight-count).<br>7. One Ribcage Undulation (two-count), one Ribcage Circle R (two-count).<br>8. One Ribcage Undulation (two-count), one Ribcage Circle L (two-count). | 1. Eight Three-Quarter Shimmies (start right).<br>2. Eight Algerian Shimmies (start right).<br>3. Four Three-Quarter Shimmies, then four Algerian Shimmies (start right).<br>4. Four Three-Quarter Shimmies while standing still and then four Shoulder Shimmies walking backward. | 1. Four Egyptian Basics forward, starting right. Four Hip Drops with Kick with left hip.<br>2. Suzy Q left, two Shuffles to the right. Repeat Suzy Q to the right, Shuffles to the left.<br>3. Four Scissor Steps with right, facing front, then four Scissor Steps with left, facing right. Repeat with right, facing back. Repeat with left, facing left.<br>4. Four Arabesques traveling forward, step on right foot, kick left, walk LR. Repeat starting left, starting right, and starting left. |

# the workout

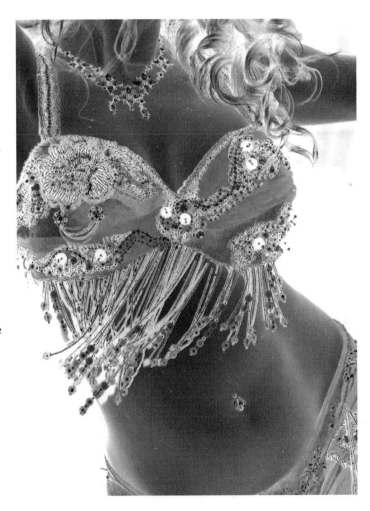

*I* recommend practicing about an hour per day, four or five times a week. The basic structure for practice sessions should begin with a warm-up, using the stretches in this book, followed by slow movements for a total of 20 to 30 minutes.

After that, bring up the energy level by practicing shimmies to drum solo music for about 10 minutes, then go into medium-tempo music with a steady but strong beat for 20 minutes, adding one or two songs that have a variety of rhythms, tempos, and accents to challenge yourself musically.

Then play a slow song to cool down while dancing with a veil. See "Make Your Own Music," earlier in the book, to create your own dance mix.

The chart on page 42 is a reasonable timeline for working on the basic movements. This sequence and timeline are also useful for any instructor teaching beginner classes. Repeat the same movements each practice day during the week.

| | MOVES | |
|---|---|---|
| **WEEK 1** | • Warm up<br>• Stretches (slow music)<br>• Slides, contractions, and circles (slow music)<br>• Shimmies—hips, shoulders, twists, and shimmy-on-toes (drum solo)<br>• Simple one-hip drops, lifts, and twists (drum solo) | • Egyptian basic, V-step, scissor step, shuffle, and Suzy Q (medium-tempo music)<br>• Experiment with improvising (varied-beat songs)<br>• *Optional:* finger cymbals—single and double time (medium-tempo music)<br>• Cool-down stretches (slow music) |
| **WEEK 2** | • Do all the movements from **Week One** and add:<br>• Undulations and wavelike movements without walking (slow music) | • Hip drops with a kick and hip crescents (medium-tempo music) |
| **WEEK 3** | • Do all the movements from **Weeks One and Two**, and add:<br>• Walking with undulations both forward and backward (slow music) | • Step together step (medium-tempo music)<br>• *Optional:* triple-time finger cymbals (no music, just get used to playing RLR slowly)<br>• Veil (slow music at the end) |
| **WEEK 4** | • Do all the movements from **Weeks One through Three**, and add:<br>• Horizontal figure eights—inside, then outside (slow music) | • *Optional:* quadruple-time finger cymbals (medium-tempo music) |
| **WEEK 5** | • Do all the movements from **Weeks One through Four**, and add:<br>• Vertical figure eights—inside, then outside (slow music) | • Turns—in place and across the floor (medium-tempo music)<br>• Arabesques (medium-tempo music) |
| **WEEK 6** | • Do the movements from **Weeks One through Five**, and add: | • Three-quarter shimmies (medium-tempo music)<br>• Up and over shimmies (medium-tempo music) |
| **WEEK 7** | Continue the same movements as **Week Six**. If you've been practicing the finger cymbals, add beledi and malfuf | rhythms. Listen to a variety of songs and try to hear these rhythms in the music. |
| **WEEK 8** | Continue the same movements as **Weeks Six and Seven**. | • Add floorwork (slow music). |

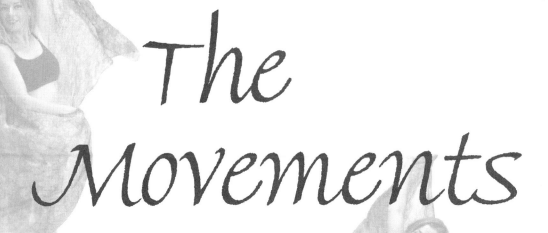

# PART 4

# The Movements

# Warm-ups

*B*efore you dance, you should always warm up your back and neck, and stretch your side muscles. Reaches, stretches, arches, and contractions are ideal warm-ups. After dancing, it is also a good idea to stretch and cool down. You can use the same warm-up routine for all workout sessions.

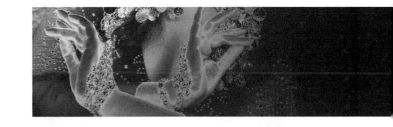

*Softness is one of the most beautiful qualities of belly dancing. It can be best achieved by relaxing and stretching.*

# Reach

*This movement lengthens the muscles along the side of your waist and helps you elongate and attain greater flexibility.*

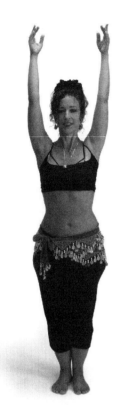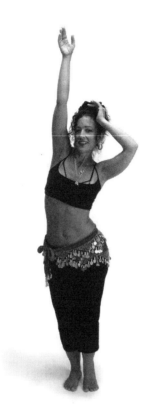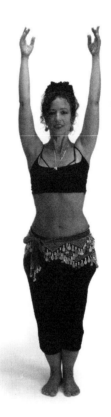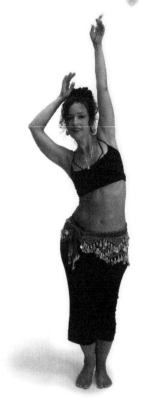

*1* Stand straight and tall, stomach in and chest lifted. Reach both arms to the ceiling.

*2* Keeping your knees and ankles together, lift your left heel, causing your left hip to lift. Bring your left arm to your head as you continue reaching toward the ceiling with your right.

*3* Return to a centered position.

*4* Still keeping your knees and ankles together, lift your right heel and hip. Reach toward the ceiling with your left arm, bringing the right arm to your head. *Return to center.*

*Repeat both sides alternately at least 10 times.*

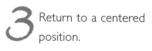

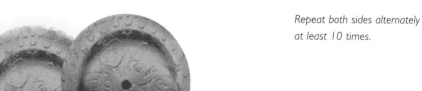

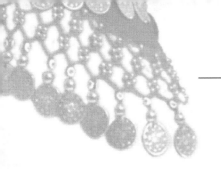

# side Stretch

*This movement stretches the waist as well as the neck. Your lower body should not move during this exercise.*

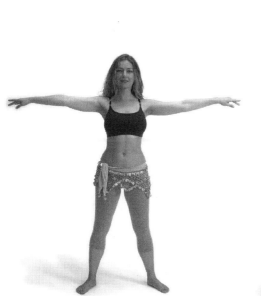

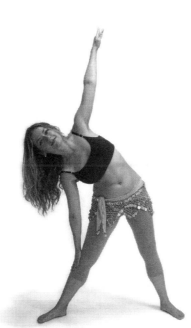

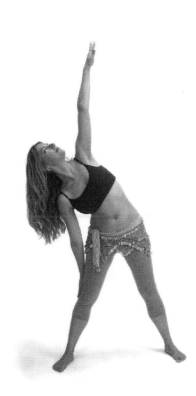

*1* Stand with your feet apart, feet grounded flat on the floor, both arms straight out to the sides.

*2* Raise your left arm and point your left hand toward the ceiling. At the same time, tilt your upper body to the right until the right hand touches your right calf.

*3* Look up toward the ceiling, then down to the floor. *Return to center before continuing the move with your left side.*

*Repeat both sides alternately at least 10 times.*

# Arch/contraction with chest

*This exercise releases tension in the upper back, improves posture, and is used in a variety of dance movements.*

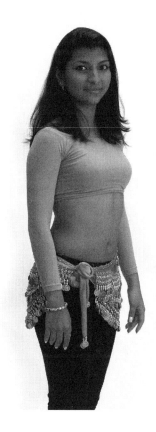 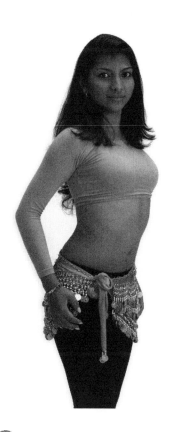 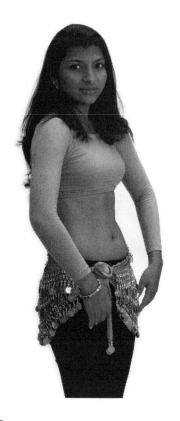

*1* Stand straight with your stomach tucked in and hips tucked under, feet grounded flat on the floor, arms relaxed at your sides.

*2* Push your chest forward, arching only your upper back, bringing your shoulder blades together. (This is an Arch.) Your lower body should not move. Keep your arms still, hips and buttocks tucked in.

*3* Cave your chest in, pushing it back and bringing the shoulders forward. (This is a Contraction.) Your lower body still should not move. Again, keep your arms still, hips and buttocks tucked in.

*Alternately arch forward and contract back at least 10 times, taking care to isolate your chest area.*

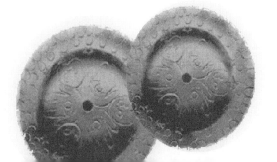

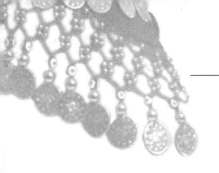

# Arch/Contraction with Pelvis

*This exercise strengthens your stomach, stretches your lower back, and is used in many belly dance movements.*

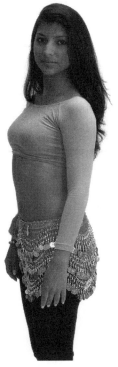

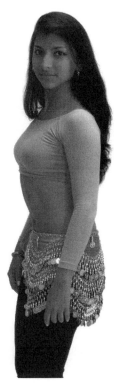

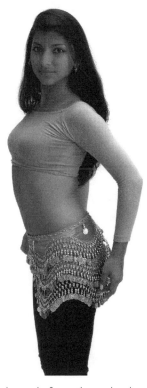

*1* Stand very straight, stomach in, chest forward, and head up, arms relaxed at your sides.

*2* Pushing in with your stomach muscles, tuck your hips under. This is a Contraction.

*3* Moving only from the waist down, push your pelvis back into an Arch, being careful not to move your upper body.

*Alternately contract and arch your pelvis at least 10 times.*

**TIP:** You can make the Contraction stronger by standing with your back to a wall and pushing every vertebra of your spine into the wall.

**warm-ups**

49

# Neck Stretch

*This movement helps release tension and prepares you for dance moves that involve the neck.*

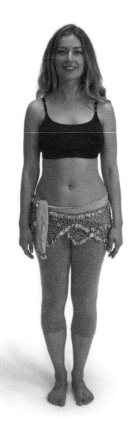

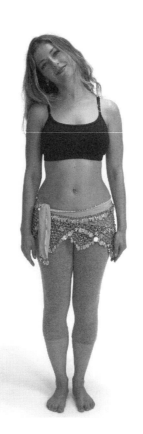

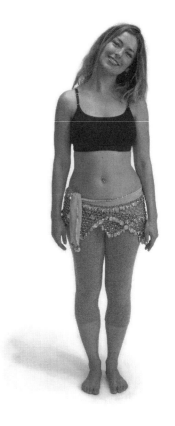

*1* Stand straight with both feet grounded flat on the floor and your arms relaxed at your sides.

*2* Drop your head to the right.

*3* Return your head to the upright position and then drop your head to the left.

*Alternate from side to side slowly several times.*

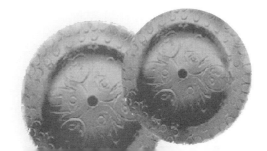

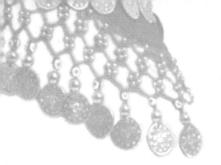

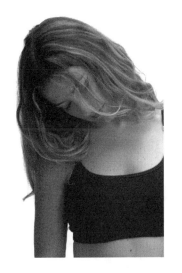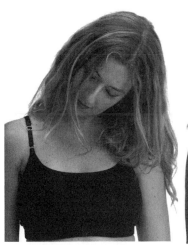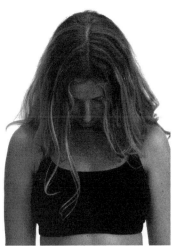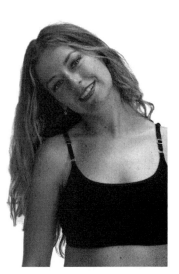

4 Bringing your chin to your neck, drop your head to the right, and from there to a diagonal right, and hold.

5 Return to center, with your chin still down to your neck, and then drop your head left, then diagonal left, and hold.

6 Return to center and drop your chin to your collarbone.

7 Alternate your head in half-circles, moving right, diagonal, center, left diagonal, and left. *Reverse directions.*

*Continue until your neck feels loose and flexible.*

# Hand Stretch

*Our hands hold a lot of tension. In belly dance, it is important that the hands be very soft and fluid, which is attained by relaxation.*

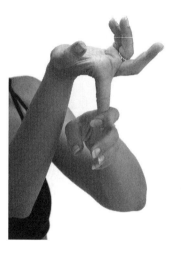 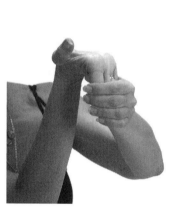 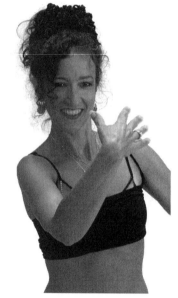 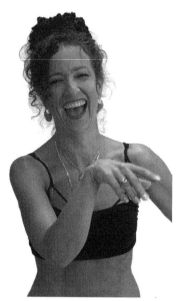

*1* With your right palm facing the ceiling, take hold of each finger with your other hand and, one at a time, bend each finger back, massaging away the tension.

*2* Bend all of your fingers back at once.

*3* Shake your hand side to side.

*4* Shake your hand up and down.

*Repeat with the left hand.*

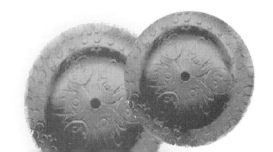

# Alphabets

*If you do these every day, your hips and upper body will become much more flexible and all the movements you learn will come easier.*

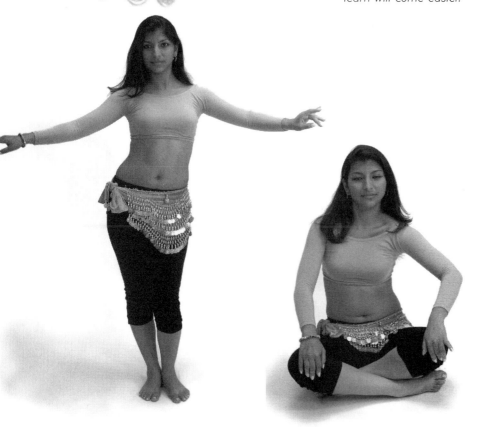

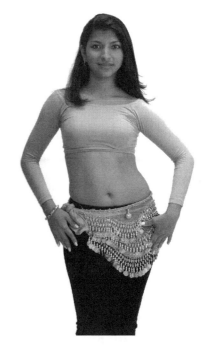

*1* **Hips:** Imagining a pen centered between your hips, write the lower-case cursive letters of the alphabet using forward, back, and side-to-side movements. Try to keep your upper body motionless as you do this.

*2* **Ribcage:** Sit cross-legged on the floor and imagine that the pen extends from the center of your chest. Again, write the lower-case cursive letters of the alphabet on the floor with the imaginary pen while maintaining your upright position.

*3* Next, try the alphabet from your ribcage again, this time standing up.

## warm-ups

# Fundamental Movements

The fundamental movements are exercises that are essential building blocks in belly dancing. This is the basic vocabulary of movement that almost all belly dance steps are built upon.

# Slow Movements

## Use Slow Music for All

The slow movements help tone your muscles and increase flexibility. They use the most muscle of all belly dance movements because they go deeper—the slower you do them, the better they tone you. Once you master slow movements, you will love them, so practice, practice, practice.

Slow movements can be divided into the following "families": Slides, Circles, Undulations, and Figure Eights.

**Slides** are isolated side-to-side movements that can be done with the head, ribcage, and hips.

**Circles** are the soft symbols of infinity and flow—no hard edges here. They can be done with the shoulders, arms, hands, ribcage, and hips.

**Undulations** are the ultimate stretch. They are wavelike movements done with the pelvis, ribcage, arms, and hands. This series of slow, sustained movements makes the muscles work deep to tone, strengthen, and stretch.

There are four different types of **Figure Eights**—*horizontal inward*, *horizontal outward*, *vertical inward*, and *vertical outward*. All are done with the hips. Highly expressive, never-ending, and flowing, Figure Eights stretch and tone the muscles of the waistline and help to make your waist smaller. The Figure Eights are isolated, so you only move from the waist down, keeping your upper body relaxed and still.

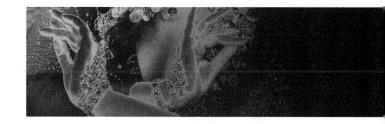

*The slow movements are the most sensual moves of the belly dance, and they are also the most difficult.*

# Head Slide

*Head Slides are gentle, isolated side-to-side stretches of the neck without twisting or moving forward or back. These made their way into belly dancing from Central Asia.*

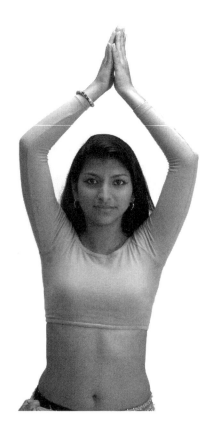 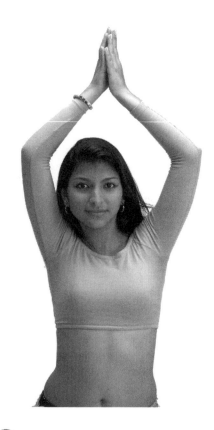 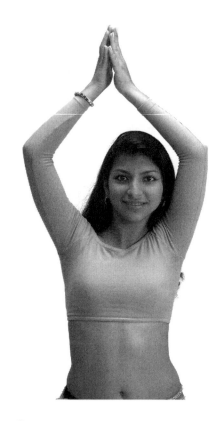

*1* Standing straight—stomach in, chest lifted, and shoulders down—bring your arms overhead and press your palms together. Look straight ahead and make sure that there is an even amount of space between your arms and the sides and top of your head.

*2* Relaxing all the muscles in the back of your neck, gently slide the head to the right. Be careful not to turn or tilt the head. Keep looking straight ahead.

*3* Slide your head to the left, continuing to look straight ahead.

*Do the Head Slide 8 times in place, then 8 times while walking forward. Do another 8 in place, then 8 times walking backward.*

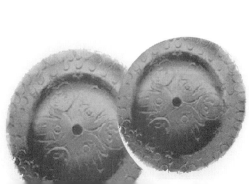

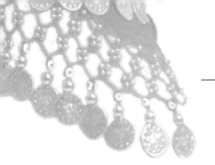

# Ribcage Slide

*Ribcage Slides are gentle, isolated side-to-side movements of the ribcage without involvement from the shoulders or hips.*

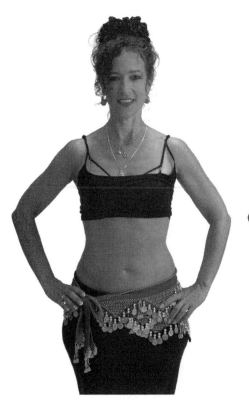 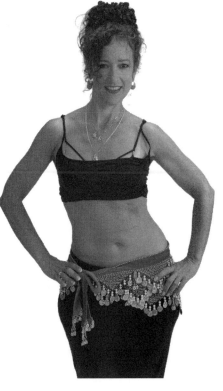 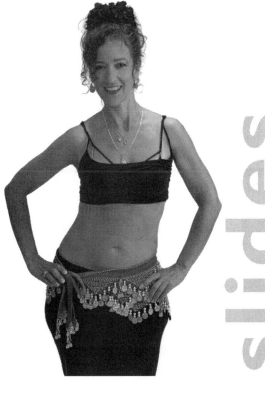

**slides**

*1* Lift your chest and keep it slightly forward from your hips, with your shoulders back, your stomach in, and your feet grounded flat on the floor.

*2* With your hands on your hips, slide your ribcage to the right. Keep your shoulders relaxed and make sure they don't move.

*3* Keeping your hands and shoulders in the same position, slide your ribcage to the left.

*Do the Ribcage Slide 8 times with your hands on your hips. Next, slowly lift your arms out to the side and slide 8 more times. Then raise your arms straight overhead and slide 8 more times.*

**TIP:** As the arms move up, you will notice different muscles being used. Lift your arms as high as you can without losing the Ribcage Slide. If you lose the movement, lower your arms a little bit. Gradually get your arms to lift higher each day.

# Hip Slide

*The easiest and most natural of the slide "family," Hip Slides stretch and tone your waistline.*

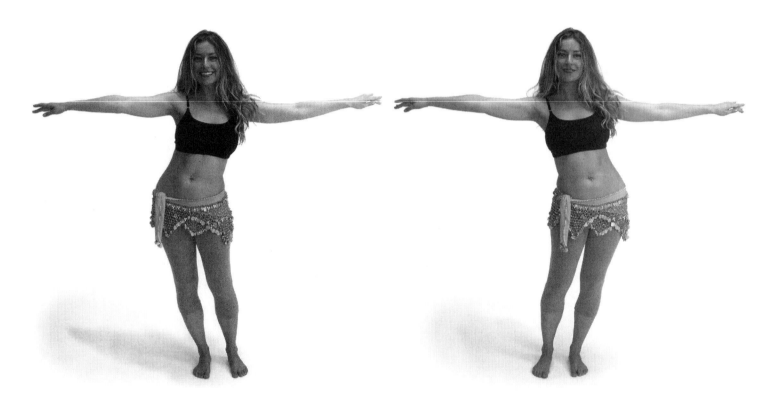

*1* Stand with your feet approximately four inches apart, knees straight but not locked. Hold your arms out to the side. Feeling the floor with your feet, shift the weight from one foot to the other, always maintaining good posture. If you look down, you should see your chest, but not your stomach or pelvis. Now slide your hips to the right without bending your knees.

*2* Keeping the same position and posture, slide your hips to the left.

*Alternating right, left, right, left, slide the hips from side to side 8 times, keeping the knees straight and feeling your weight shift from one foot to the other as you slide.*

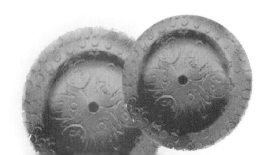

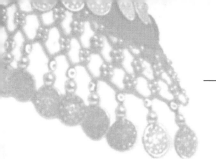

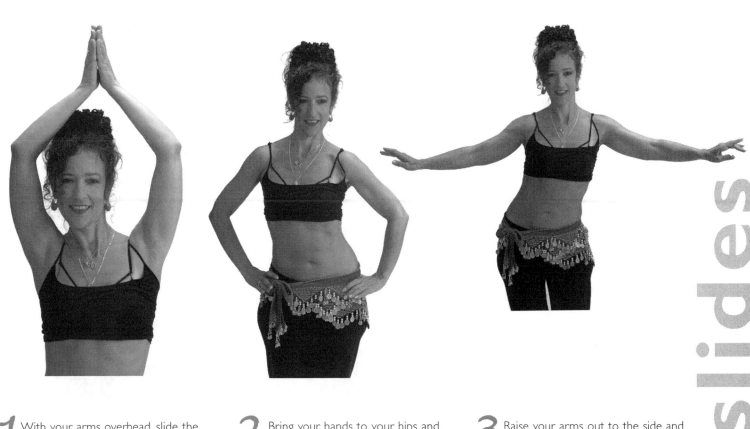

slides

*1* With your arms overhead, slide the head 8 times.

*2* Bring your hands to your hips and slide the ribcage 8 times.

*3* Raise your arms out to the side and slide your hips 8 times.

*Then do each slide—head, ribcage, and hips—4 more times.*

# Shoulder Circles

*These movements release tension in the shoulders and relax the upper back.*

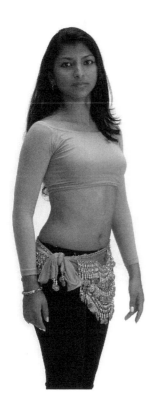

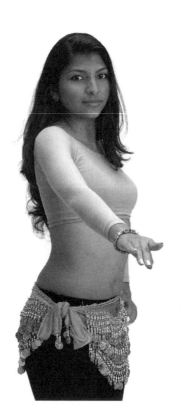

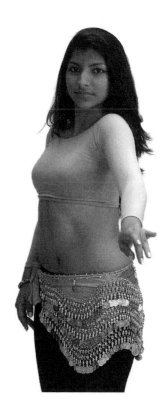

*1* Stand with good posture, feet together, chest lifted and slightly forward, and stomach pulled in. Keep your chin pulled up and keep all of your muscles relaxed.

*2* Extend your right arm to the side on a slight forward diagonal. Push your right shoulder forward, lift it up, bring it back, then down, making a full circle. *Repeat this circle 8 times.*

*3* Do the same on your left: forward, up, back, and down. *Circle the left shoulder 8 times.*

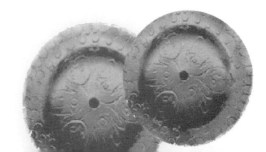

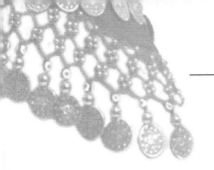

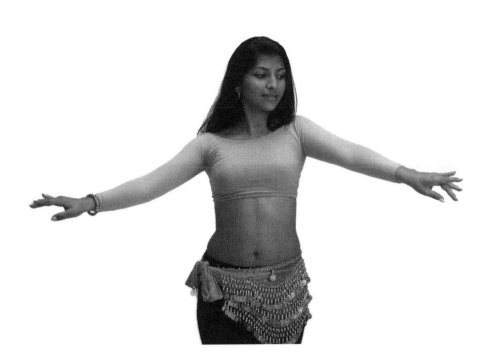

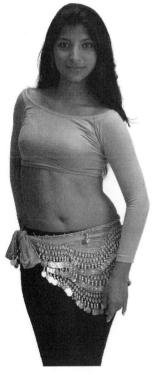

*4* Circle your right and left shoulders at the same time. The right shoulder goes forward as the left pushes back, right shoulder down as the left comes up. Left forward and right back, left down as the right comes up. *Do these Shoulder Circles 16 times.*

## In Motion

Walking while doing Shoulder Circles is beautiful and catlike. As you step forward with your left foot, circle your right shoulder; then when you step with your right foot, circle your left shoulder. Make sure that when you step forward, you put your foot flat on the floor. (If you have a cat, watch how it walks. They always step with their back legs opposite from their shoulder movements, in perfect balance.)

# Sunrise Arms

## ARM CIRCLES

*Often called Sunrise Arms and Sunset Arms, these movements stretch and elongate your waist and arms.*

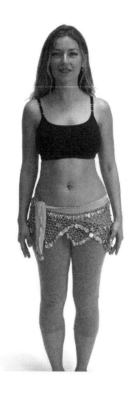

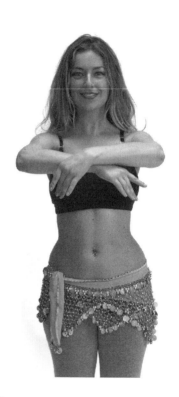

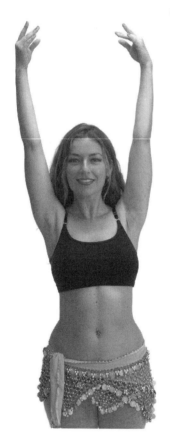

*1* Stand straight, with your stomach pulled in and chest lifted. Keep the shoulders down and relaxed and your arms down by your sides.

*2* Lifting from the elbows, cross your wrists and lift your arms to chest level.

*3* Keep pulling up with the elbows, followed by the wrists, lifting your arms straight overhead. When your arms are straight up, making sure to keep your shoulders down, stretch upward, lengthening from the waist.

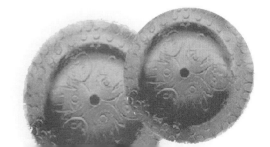

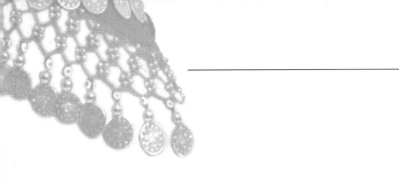

## In Motion

Take one step for each complete Sunrise; repeat 4 times.

Next, try it with two steps for each complete Sunrise—one step with your right foot as the arms come up, then a step with your left foot as the arms come down. Do this variation 4 times.

Step four times for each Sunrise: Step with your right foot as the arms come to center, then step with the left as the arms reach up. Step with the right as your arms go out to the sides, and step with the left as the arms come down. Do this 8 times, making sure you divide the movement into four equal parts to match the four steps. As you practice, work on making the Sunrise Arms flow with awareness of the four points, but do not pause at each point.

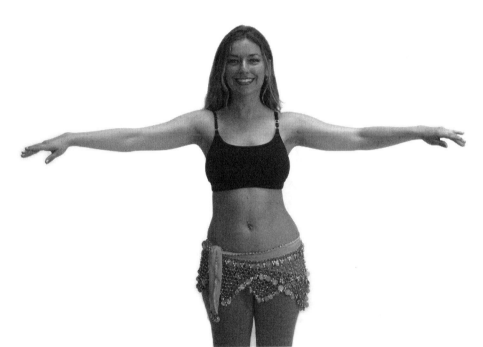

4 Lower your arms out to the sides, keeping them straight and bringing them just below shoulder level. Then lower the arms back to the sides of your hips.

*Repeat 8 times, then try it walking forward (see "In Motion").*

circles

# Sunset Arms

## ARM CIRCLES

*These are the opposite of Sunrise Arms. The move is very common in belly dance routines.*

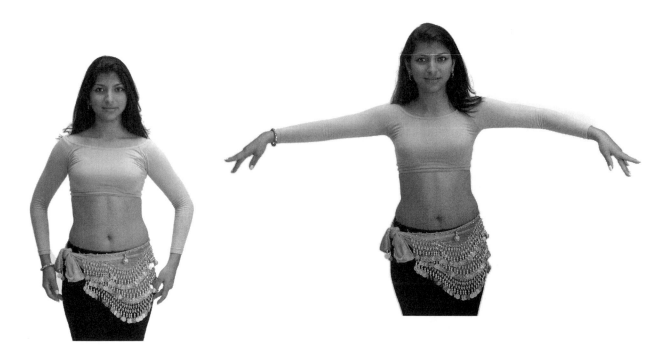

*1* Stand straight with your stomach pulled in and chest lifted. Keep your shoulders down and relaxed, and begin with your arms down.

*2* Starting with the elbows first, lift your arms straight out to the sides, slightly below shoulder level.

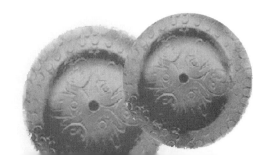

## In Motion

Try it walking backward: Take one step back for each complete Sunset Arm circle. Repeat 4 times. Now try it with two steps. Starting with your arms down, step back with your right foot and bring your arms out to the sides and up overhead. Step back with your left foot and bring the arms down, crossing them over your chest and down. Repeat 4 times.

Now step four times for each Sunset. Step with your right as your arms go out to the sides, then with your left as your arms come up overhead; step with your right as the arms cross over your chest, and step with your left as your arms come down. Repeat this four-step Sunset Arm circle 8 times.

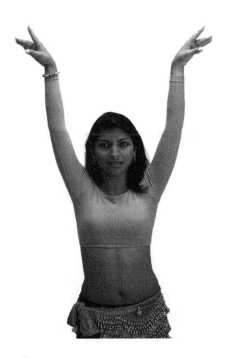

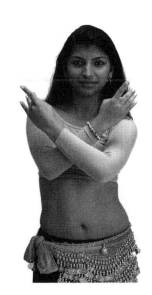

3 Continue to lift with the elbows, bringing the arms straight up. Keep your shoulders down and relaxed while lifting from the chest and lengthening the sides of the waist.

4 Lower the arms, using the elbows and crossing the wrists, until they reach the level of your chest. Then drop your arms to the sides of your hips.

*Repeat the Sunset Arms 8 times, making them flow through the four positions.*

circles

# Hand Circles—Outside

*The hands are one of the most expressive parts of belly dancing, and one of the most important ways of using them is to make circles. Exercising and stretching your hands releases tension—very important in a society where we use our hands excessively to type on computers and tightly grasp the steering wheel of our car in aggravating*

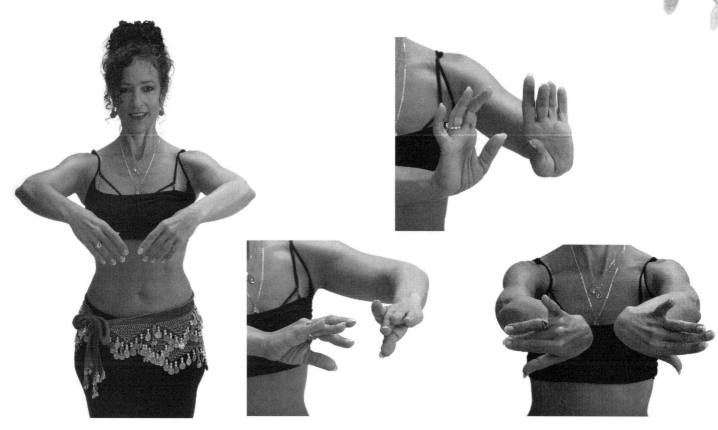

**1** Stand straight, chest lifted, stomach in, and shoulders down. Bring your arms to slightly below chest level, in a rounded position as if you are hugging a big beach ball.

**2** Position your hands in a "C" shape, connecting your thumb and middle finger with an invisible strand of energy about two inches long. All the other fingers should be slightly lifted away from the middle finger.

**3** Maintaining the "C" shape, bend your hands back at the wrists so they face away from you.

**4** Twist your wrists so your hands face out to the sides.

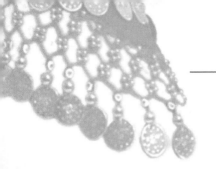

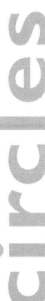

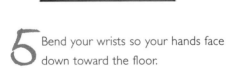

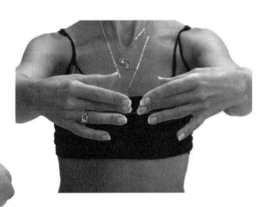

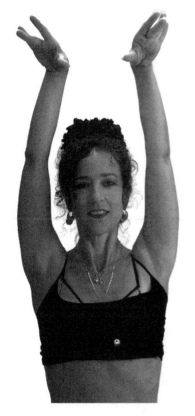

**5** Bend your wrists so your hands face down toward the floor.

**6** Bring your hands in to face each other, as the palms of your hands face your chest.

*Repeat these circles, carefully passing through all four positions, smoothing out all the rough edges until they form complete circles. Repeat the Hand Circles 8 times, keeping your arms in the rounded position.*

*Change position so your arms are straight out to the sides, and repeat the Hand Circles 8 more times.*

*Bring the arms straight overhead and repeat the Hand Circles 8 more times.*

# Hand Circles—inside

*This inside circle is more dramatic, though less common, than the outside circle in belly dancing. It is often seen in ethnic Persian and Gypsy dances and gives added stretch and flexibility to the hands and wrists.*

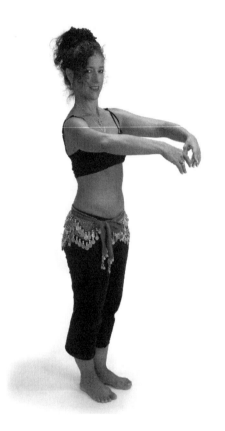

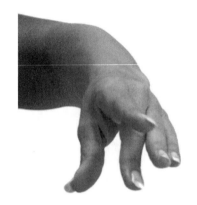

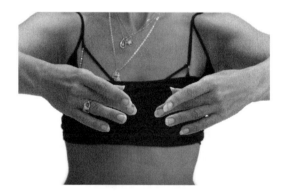

*1* Stand straight, chest lifted, stomach in, and shoulders down. Bring your arms to slightly below chest level, in a rounded position as if you are hugging a big beach ball.

*2* Position your hands in a "C" shape, connecting your thumb and middle finger with an invisible strand of energy about two inches long. All the other fingers should be slightly lifted away from the middle finger.

*3* Maintaining the "C" shape, bring your hands in to face each other, as the palms of your hands face your chest.

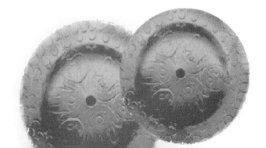

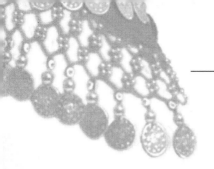

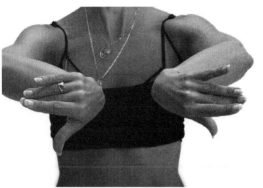

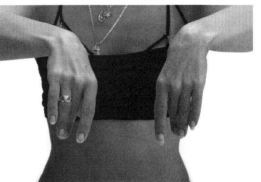

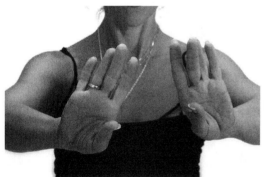

4 Bend your wrists so your hands face down.

5 Twist your wrists so your hands face the floor and out to the sides.

6 Bend your hands back at the wrists so they face away from you.

*Repeat these circles, carefully passing through all four positions, smoothing out all the rough edges until they form complete circles. Repeat the Hand Circles 8 times, keeping your arms in the rounded position.*

*Extend your arms straight out to the sides and repeat the Hand Circles 8 times.*

*Raise your arms straight overhead and circle your hands 8 more times.*

# Ribcage Circles

*Convincing the ribcage to move is one of the harder parts of belly dancing. Don't feel discouraged if the Ribcage Circle doesn't come right away. Give it two to four weeks of gentle practice because we store a lot of tension in our upper bodies. Practicing the alphabet (see page 53) with your ribcage daily will speed up the process.*

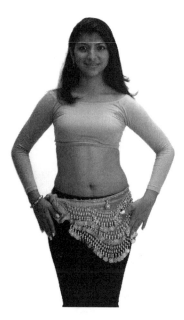 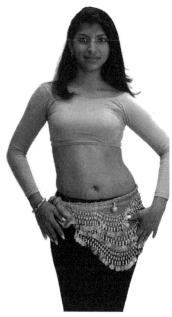 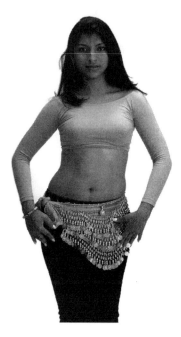 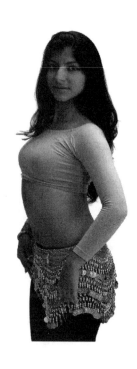

*1* Stand straight, stomach in and chest lifted, with your feet grounded flat on the floor. Place your hands on your hips.

*2* Without moving your lower body, gently slide your ribcage to the right.

*3* Slide your ribcage to the left.

*Alternate right and left slides 8 times.*

*4* Look at yourself in the mirror from the side. Check your posture before continuing. Keeping your stomach in, push your chest forward. Take care not to move from the waist down.

**TIP:** If you find it difficult to isolate your upper body and not move your hips, practice the Ribcage Circle sitting on the floor cross-legged with your hands on your knees. Then stand up when you feel more comfortable. When you are comfortable circling your ribcage while standing with your hands on your hips, try it with your arms out to the sides, then with your arms straight up overhead.

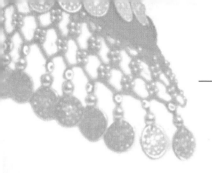

## Putting It Together

Make this sequence of movements into a circle: slide to the right, arch to the front, slide to the left, and contract to the back. Circle your ribcage to the left 8 times, each time smoothing out the rough edges to make the movement soft and circular, not angular.

Change the direction of your Ribcage Circle and go to the right: slide to the left, arch front, slide right, and contract to the back. Circle to the right 8 times.

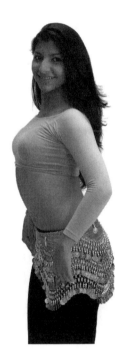

5 Contract your chest, leaning slightly back and caving the chest in, shoulders forward.

6 *Push your chest forward and back 8 times in an Arch and Contraction,* like the ones you did while stretching at the beginning of your workout. Concentrate on isolating your movement, moving only your upper back and chest and keeping the knees, hips, and shoulders still.

# Medium Hip Circles

*Medium-size Hip Circles stretch and tone your waistline and stomach muscles. They are fun and easy to do, and they fit many types of music.*

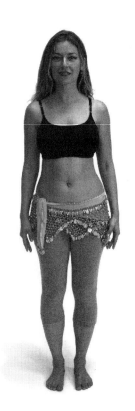

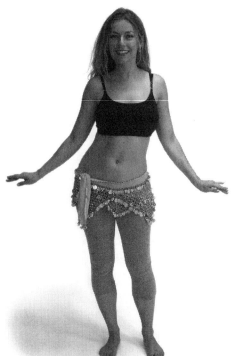

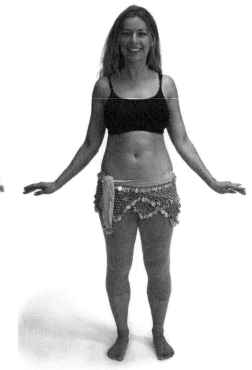

*1* Stand with your feet a few inches apart, keeping your knees straight but not locked. Avoid moving your upper body during this exercise.

*2* Slide your hips to the right.

*3* Bring your hips to the front and center.

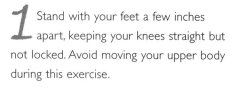

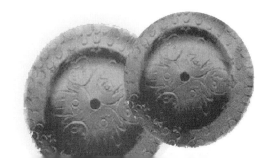

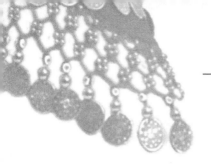

## Putting It Together

Make these four movements into a circle, sliding right, pushing center-front, sliding left, and pushing center-back. Practice maintaining a circular shape and smoothing out all the rough edges. Circle your hips to the left 8 times.

Change the direction and circle your hips to the right. Start by sliding your hips to the left, pushing center-front, sliding right, and pushing center-back. Repeat 8 times.

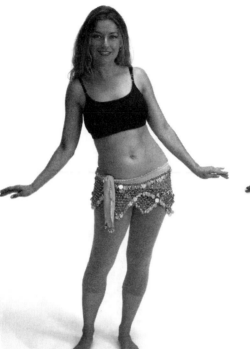

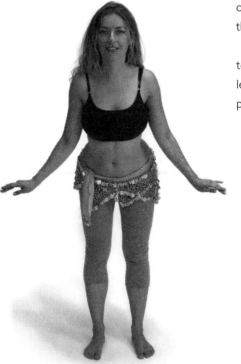

4 Slide your hips to the left.

5 Push your hips to the back and center.

*After circling your hips 8 times to the left and 8 times to the right, do it to the left 4 more times, then to the right 4 times. Then go left 2 times, right 2 times, left 2 more times and right 2 more times.*

circles

# Small Hip Circles

These are a little more difficult than the medium circles, but they really tone your stomach and stretch your lower back. Small Hip Circles look great, and when you master them your friends will say, "How do you do that? It looks hard."

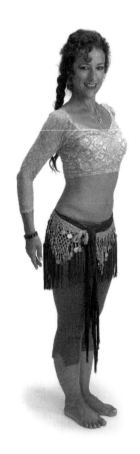

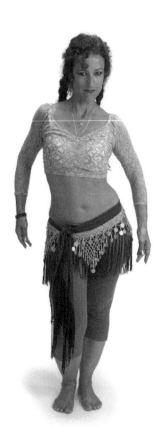

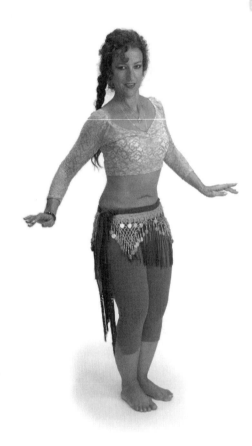

*1* Stand with your feet together, stomach in, chest lifted and slightly forward, hips tucked under, and knees straight but not locked.

*2* Switch your hips from side to side by bending and straightening the knees, alternating first one and then the other. Notice that this is different from the slide because the hips go up and down instead of straight out to the sides. *Alternate sides 8 times for practice.*

*3* Contract your pelvis. Pull your stomach in and tuck your hips way under, while keeping the chest lifted and forward. Bend the knees softly.

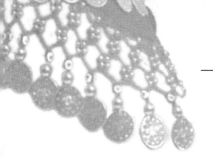

## Putting It Together

Make a Small Hip Circle to the left: Bend your left knee (keeping the right knee straight) and bring your right hip to the side and up; bend both knees as you contract into the center; straighten the left knee, keeping the right bent, which brings your left hip to the side; and straighten both knees as you arch back to the center. Repeat the Small Hip Circle 8 times, each time strengthening your contraction and bringing the stomach in more and more.

Change the direction and do your Small Hip Circle to the right. Starting with your left hip: side, contract to the center, right hip side, then arch back and center. Repeat 8 times.

## Spiral Variation

This variation takes you from medium to small Hip Circles. Begin with a Medium Hip Circle to the left, and gradually make it smaller until it becomes a Small Hip Circle. Repeat in the opposite direction, starting with a Medium Hip Circle and making it gradually smaller until it becomes a Small Hip Circle.

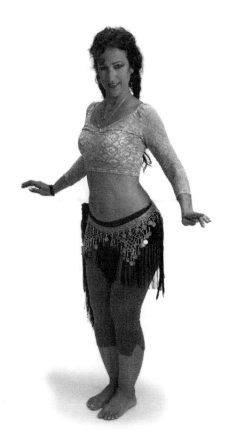

4 Arch your lower back. Straighten your knees and stretch your buttocks up and back. *Alternate this contraction and arch 8 times.*

circles

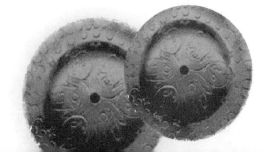

# Pelvic undulation

*Smooth out the four parts of the Undulation to make a smooth, wavelike motion. It is very important to isolate and use only your lower body, while keeping the chest still and lifted, shoulders back and relaxed.*

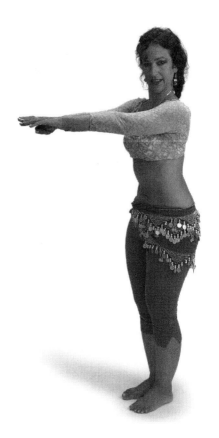 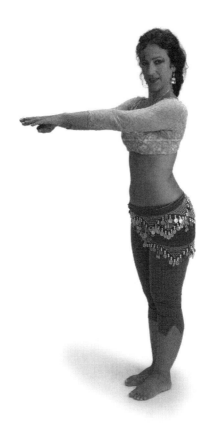 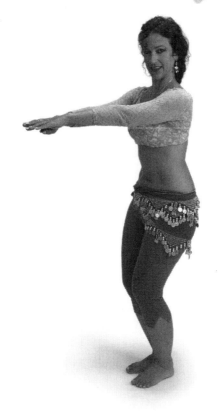

*1* **PELVIC UNDULATION PREPARATION:** Stand tall, with your knees straight and chest lifted. Tuck your hips under in a contraction. Push your stomach in against your spine by tightening your stomach muscles. Meanwhile, your lower back receives an intense stretch. If you are doing the contraction correctly, when you look down, you should only see your chest, not your pelvis or hips.

*2* Keeping your knees straight, arch your lower back by pushing your buttocks up and back, keeping the upper body relaxed and perfectly still. *Contract and arch your pelvis 8 times*, focusing a lot of energy on the contraction and utilizing the stomach muscles.

*3* Bend your knees and, keeping them bent, *contract and arch your pelvis 8 times*.

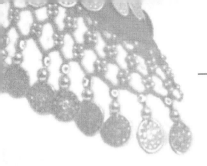

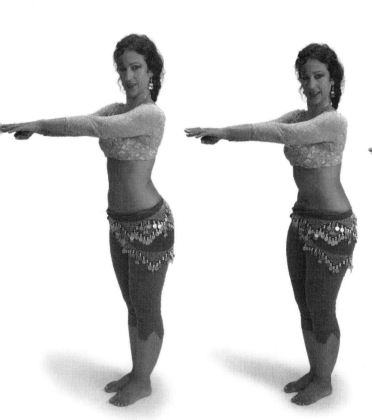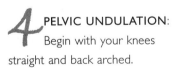

**4** **PELVIC UNDULATION**: Begin with your knees straight and back arched.

**5** Keeping your knees straight, contract your pelvis in.

**6** Holding your pelvis in, bend both knees, but do not lose the contraction.

**7** Keeping your knees bent, arch your back.

*Practice the undulation 16 times before moving on.*

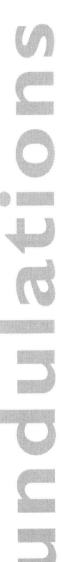

# camel walk

The Camel Walk means walking with the Pelvic Undulation. It is actually easier to walk and undulate than it is to undulate in place. Imagine that you are slowly undulating across a sandy desert. The key to coordinating the walk with the undulation is your feet.

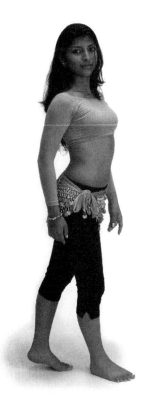
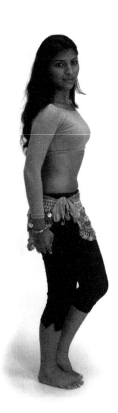
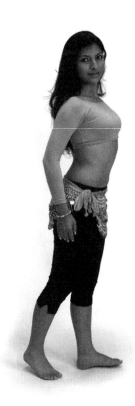
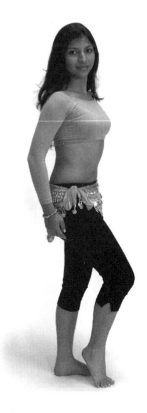

*1* Take a small step forward, placing your right foot flat on the floor. As you do this, arch your lower back. The left heel should be lifted.

*2* Drag your left foot to meet the right, keeping only the ball of your foot on the floor, ankles together. Contract your pelvis.

*3* Take a small step forward, placing your left foot flat on the floor. As you do this, arch your lower back. The right heel should be lifted.

*4* Drag your right foot to meet the left, keeping only the ball of your foot on the floor, ankles together. Contract your pelvis.

*Repeat this step, using the stepping and dragging with the arch and contraction 16 times, while doing the Camel Walk in a circle around the room.*

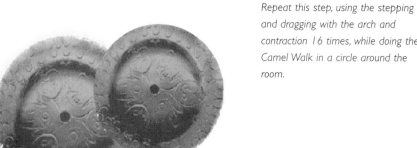
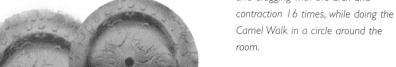

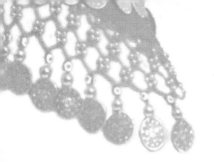

# ribcage undulation

*The contractions of the upper body release tension in your upper back and behind the shoulder blades. This undulation also strengthens and stretches your stomach muscles.*

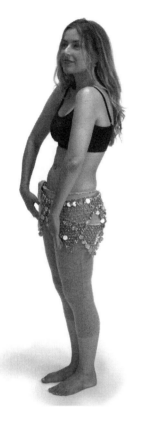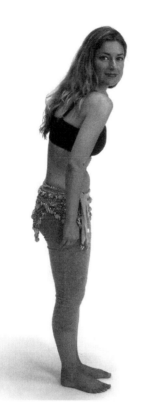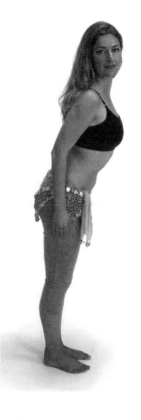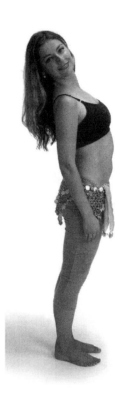

*1* Begin by standing straight, keeping your knees straight and stomach tucked in. Contract your chest, caving it inward, rounding your back, and leaning back. You are only using your upper body, so your knees, hips, and pelvis do not move. Your shoulders, neck, and arms are relaxed and also do not move.

*2* Staying contracted, lean forward.

*3* Push your chest forward into an arch.

*4* Lift the chest up and arch back. The Ribcage Undulation uses the four actions in a smooth motion: contract back, lean forward with the contraction, push forward with the arch, and arch up and back.

*Repeat the Ribcage Undulation 16 times.*

**TIP:** If you have trouble keeping your lower body from moving, you can sit cross-legged and do the Ribcage Undulation until you feel comfortable, then stand up and try again.

# Snake Arms

The Snake Arms movement gives your arms a workout and helps get rid of the sagging underarm muscles that plague so many women. We begin with both arms at the same time. I call these "Eagle Arms," but they are actually preparation for Snake Arms.

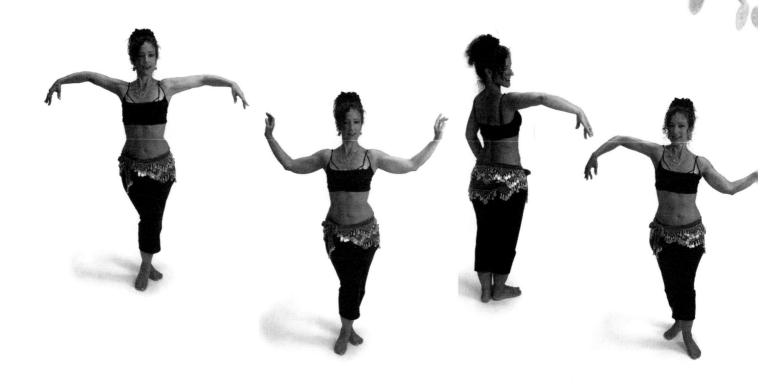

*1* With your palms facing inward, arms outstretched away from your body, lift the elbows, then the wrists, and then the hands, like wings.

*2* Keeping the arms outstretched to the sides, drop the elbows, wrists, then hands. *Lift and drop, like you are flapping wings, 8 times.*

*3* To make the Eagle Arms into Snake Arms, merely lift one arm at a time. Start with your right arm, lifting the elbow, wrist, then hand. When you can go no higher, drop your elbow, wrist, and hand. Do the same with your left arm. *Alternate the left and right arms 8 times each side.*

*4* To make this movement very snakelike, do both arms simultaneously, in opposition. Lift the right elbow as the left comes down, then lift the left elbow as the right comes down. *Repeat these 8 times with each arm.*

**TIP:** Keep in mind that in dance, the arms do not begin at the shoulder socket but extend all the way back to the muscles behind the shoulder blades, so you must think of those muscles when lifting your arms. That will make the arms feel lighter.

# *Persian Arms*

*This undulatory movement is easier than Snake Arms, but equally beautiful.*

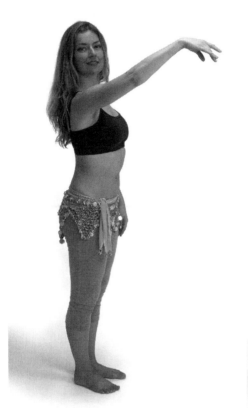 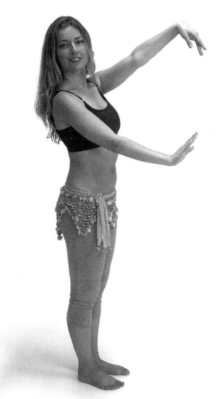

*1* Begin with both arms down in front of your thighs. Lift your right arm, elbow first, then your wrist, keeping the palm of your hand facing your body until the arm comes all the way up.

*2* As you lower the right arm, palm facing away from you, lift your left arm, palm facing you, elbow first, then wrist and hand. The hands should pass next to each other, right facing out and left facing in, until the left arm is up and the right is down.

*Repeat, lifting the right arm from the elbow, palm facing in, lowering the left arm, palm facing out. Alternate the right and left arms, making sure they meet in the middle. Repeat this movement 8 times with each arm.*

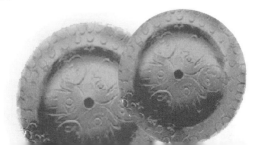

# Hand Waves

*This movement is an excellent stretch for your hands and helps release tension built up after a long day at work.*

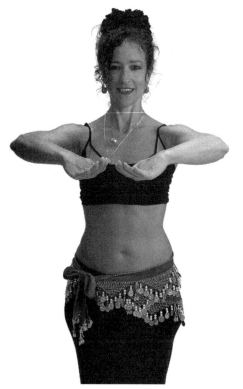
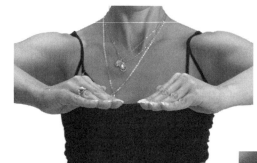
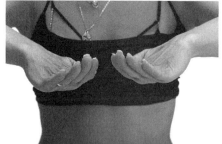

*1* Begin by standing straight, arms rounded in front of you, Keeping all of your fingers together and the thumbs next to your hands, push the balls of your hands down, stretching the fingers up and as far back as possible.

*2* Cup your hands, lifting the balls of your hands and bringing the fingers slightly downward.

*3* Push the balls of your hands down again, this time lifting your fingers first, one knuckle at a time, until they are straight up, pushing the ball of your hand down at the same time. *Repeat the Hand Wave 16 times.*

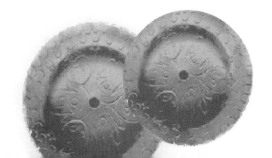

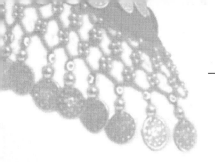

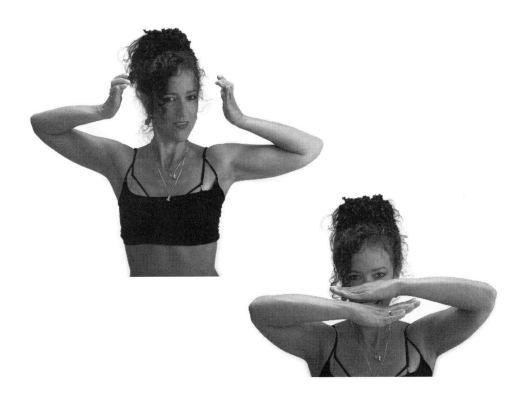

**4** **RAINING HAND WAVES:** Lift your arms high overhead, palms facing each other. Slowly bring the arms down alongside your body as you do Hand Waves. Make 8 Hand Waves as your hands descend from overhead all the way down to the level of your hips. Bring the arms up and repeat the 8 Hand Waves as you lower your arms. *Do this combination 4 times.*

**5** **THE VEILED LADY:** Cross your hands under your eyes as if they are a veil. Keep your elbows lifted and slowly open your arms as you do 8 Hand Waves. Cross again and repeat the 8 Hand Waves, opening the arms. *Do this 8 times.*

undulations

# Turkish Eight

## HORIZONTAL INWARD FIGURE EIGHT

*The name "Turkish Eight" is for identification purposes only since this Figure Eight exists throughout the Middle East, not just in Turkey. Imagine that you are making an "X" with your hips, and then connect the lines and make it look like an eight.*

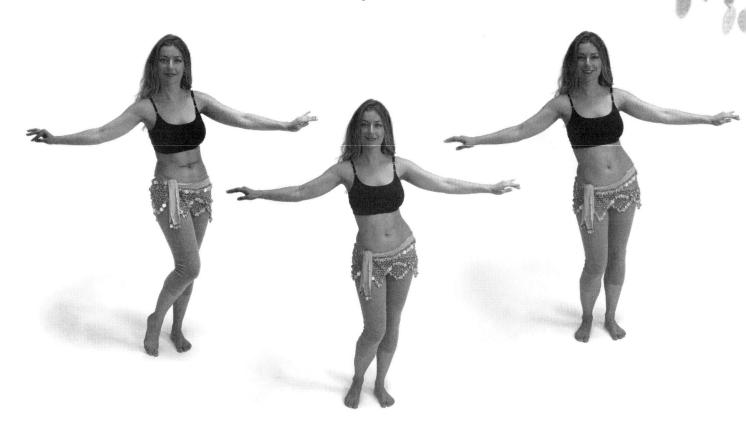

*1* Twist your right hip to the front, keeping the left foot flat and right heel lifted. Twist from the waist, but keep your chest lifted and facing forward, stomach in.

*2* Shift the weight from your right foot to your left foot, pushing the right hip diagonally back from the right to the left without changing the foot position.

*3* Set the right heel down so both feet are grounded flat on the floor.

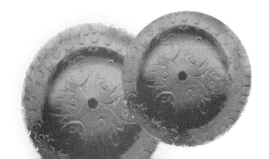

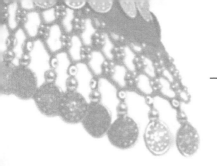

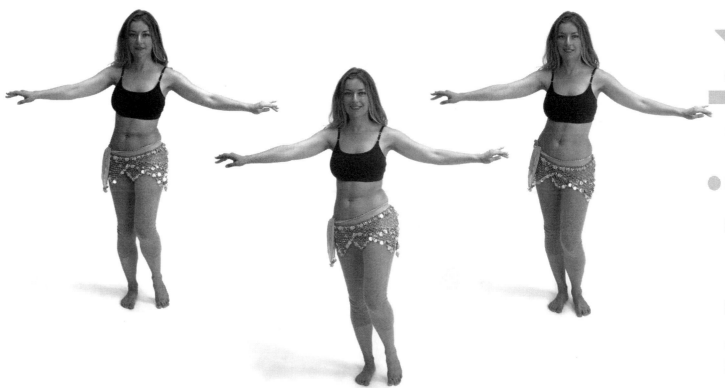

4 Lift the left heel as you twist the left hip to the front, keeping the right foot flat and left heel lifted. Twist from the waist, but keep your chest lifted and facing forward, stomach in.

5 Shift the weight from your left to your right foot, pushing the left hip diagonally back from the left to the right without changing the foot position.

6 Set the left heel down so both feet are flat on the floor. Merge the movements together to make a smooth Figure Eight.

*Repeat the Figure Eight 16 times.*

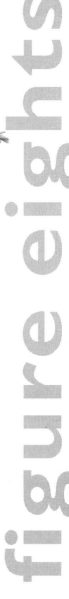

figure eights

# Egyptian Eight

**HORIZONTAL OUTWARD FIGURE EIGHT**

*The name "Egyptian Eight" is for identification purposes only since this movement exists in many Arabic countries as well as in Turkey and Iran.*

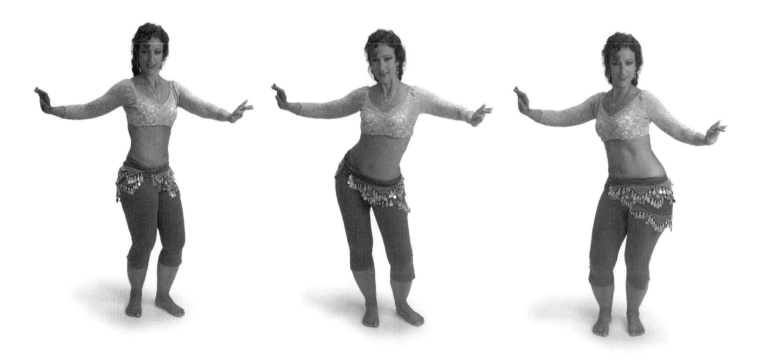

*1* Twist your right hip to the front.

*2* Carefully draw a circle to the outside with your right hip until it is facing diagonally back. Feel that your weight is still on your right foot.

*3* Shift your weight to the left foot and cross your hip to the left diagonal front.

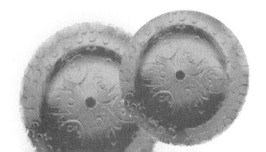

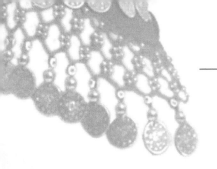

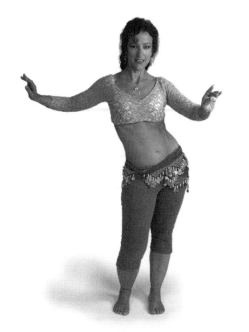
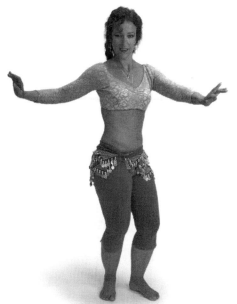

4 Draw a circle to the outside with your left hip until it is facing diagonally back, keeping your weight on the left foot.

5 Shift your weight to the right foot and cross the hip to the right diagonal front. Merge the movements together to make a smooth Figure Eight.

*Repeat this horizontal outward Figure Eight 16 times.*

**TIP:** With this Figure Eight, it is very important to keep your feet flat on the floor. Relax your whole body and imagine that you are drawing all of your energy from the earth. Imagine that you have really big hips and you are proud of them. Bend your knees and sink your weight down. Don't forget your posture. Keep your stomach in and be careful not to arch your back.

# Sway

**VERTICAL INWARD FIGURE EIGHT**

*When you do the Sway, imagine that you're between two panes of glass—your hips cannot move forward or back, only side to side.*

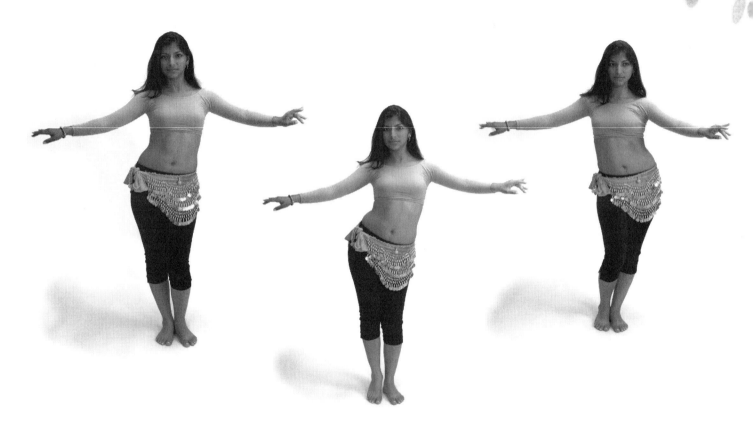

*1* Stand straight, stomach in, chest lifted. Keep both feet flat on the floor as you push your right hip out to the side.

*2* Lift your right heel as your right hip comes up.

*3* Cross the right hip diagonally down to the left, shifting your weight to your left foot as you push your left hip out to the side. Both feet are now flat again.

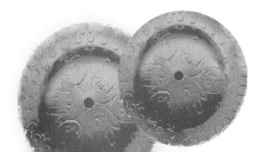

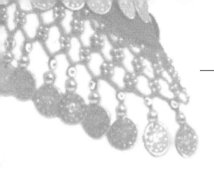

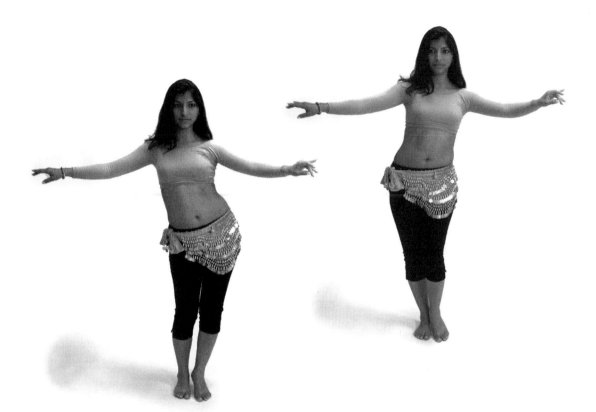

**4** Lift your left heel as the left hip comes up.

**5** Cross your left hip diagonally down to the right, shifting your weight to your right foot as you push your right hip out to the side once again. Both feet are now flat.

*Repeat the Sway 16 times.*

# Maya

## VERTICAL OUTWARD FIGURE EIGHT

*This movement was named after a dancer in the 1960s who became famous for doing it flat-footed. This was her signature movement. Doing it properly takes time and practice. We begin by doing the Maya with lifted heels; the more advanced version of the Maya is flat-footed, keeping both heels down at all times, and using only your knees to lift and lower the hips.*

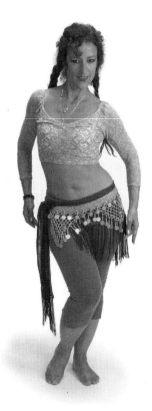 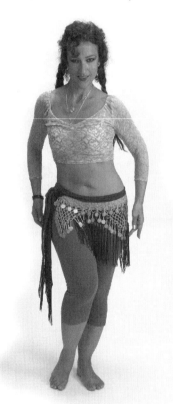 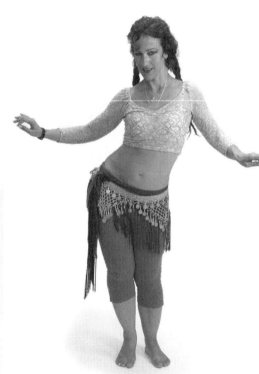

*1* With both feet flat on the floor, push your left hip out as you put your weight on your left foot.

*2* Lift the right hip up directly under your ribcage as the left hip remains out to the left, in what is known as a "sideways contraction." The right heel comes up as well.

*3* With a circular motion, arc the right hip up and over to the right, placing your right heel down, right hip out, and both feet flat, weight on your right foot.

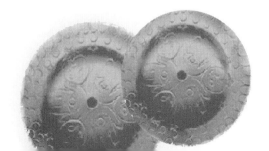

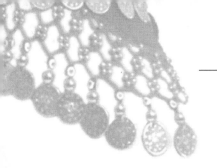

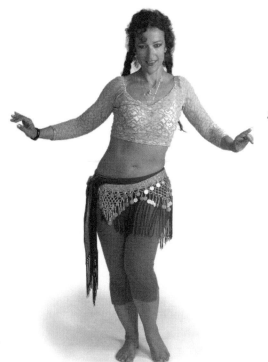

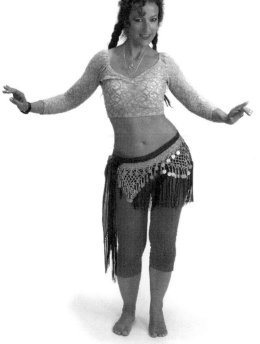

4 Lift the left hip up in the "sideways contraction," directly under your ribcage, as the right hip remains out to the right. The left heel comes up as well.

5 With a circular motion, arc the left hip up and over to the left, placing your left heel down, right hip out, and both feet flat, weight on your left foot.

*Repeat the Maya 16 times.*

# shimmies

## Use Drum Solo Music

**F**ast movements are composed of **Shimmies**, the cardio-vascular, calorie-burning part of belly dancing. Here we'll cover both basic shimmies and the more complex Up and Over (Algerian) Shimmy and Three-Quarters Shimmy. Shimmies are done with the hips or the shoulders, but never at the same time. They are usually done to the beat of a drum called a dumbek. More often than not, the arms are held at waist level or below because the shimmies use an earthy energy.

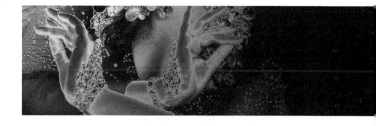

If I feel like I can't

shimmy any longer,

I look up at the stars,

take a deep breath,

and my shimmy

gets stronger.

# Hip Shimmy

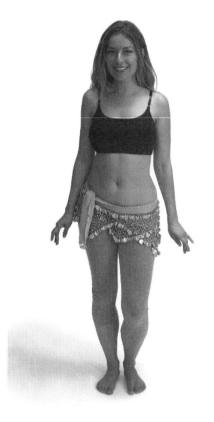

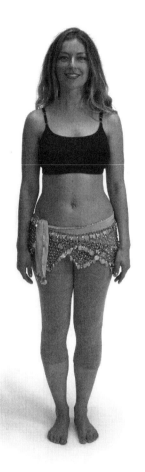

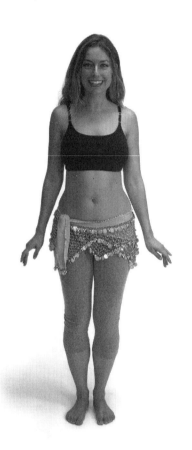

*1* Relax your knees and hips, and keep both feet flat on the floor throughout this movement. Keep both heels glued to the ground at all times.

*2* Bend your right knee. Do not lift your heel from the floor.

*3* Straightening your right knee, bend your left knee. Do not lift your heel from the floor.

*Repeat Shimmy for 16 counts. Start slow, then gradually increase the speed.*

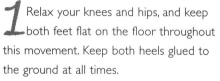

**TIP:** When you freeze up, that means you are shimmying faster than you are ready for, so simply slow down. The faster you go, the more you have to relax. Do not force your hips to move; if you relax, the knees will cause them to move up and down.

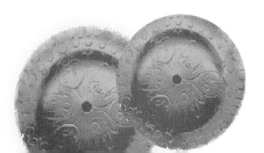

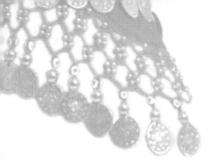

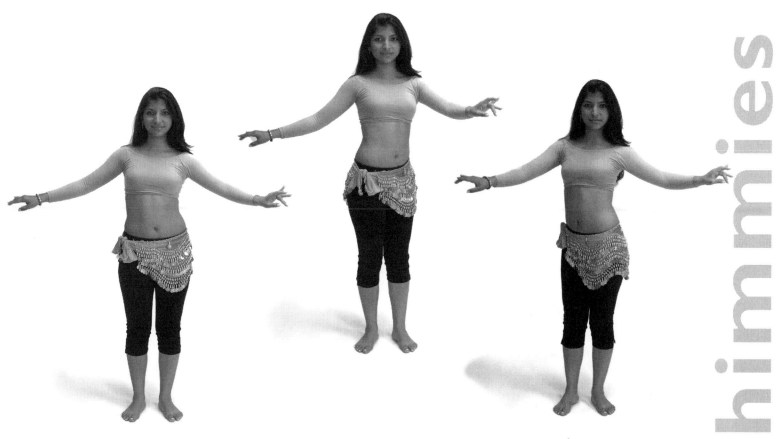

*1* Keep your knees straight and your feet slightly apart. Both feet are flat on the floor. Do not lift the heels.

*2* Twist your hips, right hip forward and left hip back.

*3* Twist your hips the other way, left hip forward and right hip back.

*Twist 16 counts, then Shimmy 16 counts; repeat several times.*

**TIP:** Alternate your hips, gradually building up speed. Don't forget to breathe. If you get a muscle cramp in your stomach, relax and take a few deep breaths.

**shimmies**

# Hip Shimmy on Toes

*Shimmying on your toes from one end of the room to the other is very aerobic and builds strong leg muscles.*

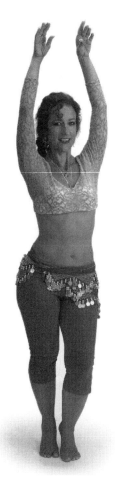

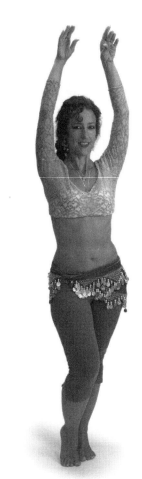

*1* Keeping your legs together, rise up onto the balls of your feet.

*2* Scoot forward. Use the same knee action as the Hip Shimmy, alternately bending and straightening.

*Repeat until you've shimmied across the room.*

**TIP:** Gradually build up speed, keeping your toes on the floor and your heels up. By scooting and not lifting either foot completely off the ground, your Shimmy will be silent. It should not sound like you are stomping, but should be a delicate glide with lots of hip action.

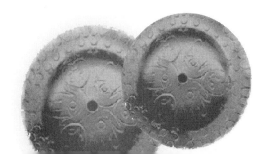

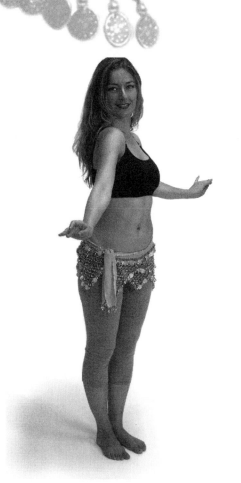

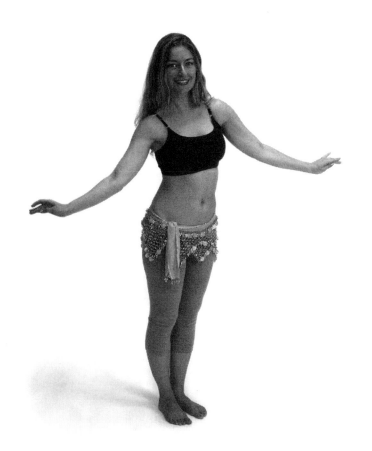

**shimmies**

*1* Holding your arms gently sloping to waist level, push the right shoulder forward as the left goes back.

*2* Reverse shoulder positions, pushing the left shoulder forward as the right goes back. Start slowly, being careful not to move the arms and hands.

*Repeat the alternation, gradually increasing the speed as you get comfortable with the movement. Shimmy your shoulders for one minute.*

**TIP:** Keeping your arms and hands relaxed will allow them to be still and help you isolate the shoulders. You can practice Shoulder Shimmies with your hands resting on a table or against a wall until you get used to moving only your shoulders.

# up and over shimmy

*This movement is often called the "Algerian shimmy," although it is done throughout the Middle East and is more popular in Egypt than in Algeria. This Shimmy must be learned and practiced slowly, making it a staccato movement. Once you get used to it and it's ingrained in your body, increase the speed so that it looks like a Shimmy.*

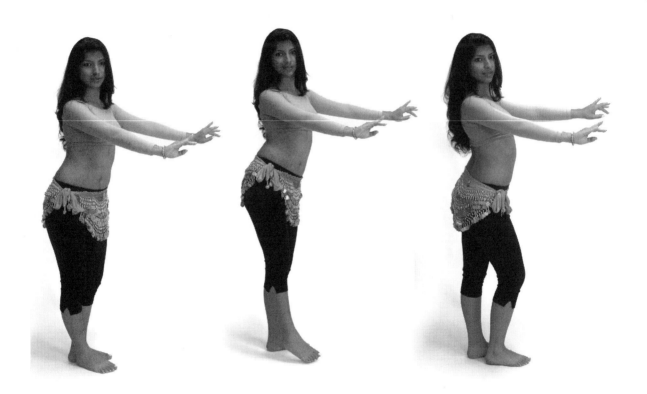

**1–3** Start by circling the right hip (1) back, (2) up, lifting the right foot as the hip comes up, over, and (3) down, and setting the right foot down flat as the hip comes down. *Circle the right hip a few times to get used to the feeling. Then switch sides.*

## In Motion

You may notice that the feet want to go pigeon-toed or cross over as you step. Neither of these is correct. Try the following walk separately from the hip movement:

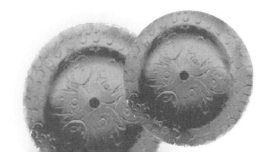

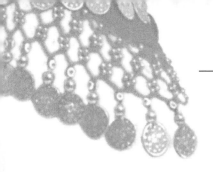

## Putting It Together

Put the walk and the hip movement together. Lift each hip at the same time the opposite heel lifts and twists. When you put your foot down flat, the same hip is forward and down. Alternate right foot and hip, left foot and hip. Gradually build up speed. Do this 32 times.

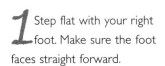

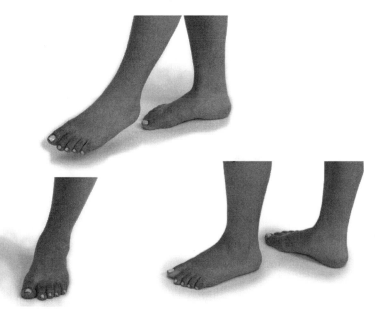

*1* Step flat with your right foot. Make sure the foot faces straight forward.

*2* Twist the left heel inward with a slight lift.

*3* Step flat with your left foot, again making sure the foot faces straight forward.

*4* Twist the right heel inward with a slight lift.

*Try this walk, alternating feet a few times, and then coordinate it with the hip movement.*

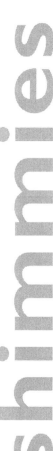

shimmies

99

# Three-Quarters Shimmy

*Like the Up and Down Shimmy, this must be learned and practiced slowly. You can also use the slow version in your dancing. Once you get used to it and it is ingrained in your body, increase the speed so that it looks like a Shimmy. The Three-Quarters Shimmy involves three moves but the music allows for four, so hold the fourth beat.*

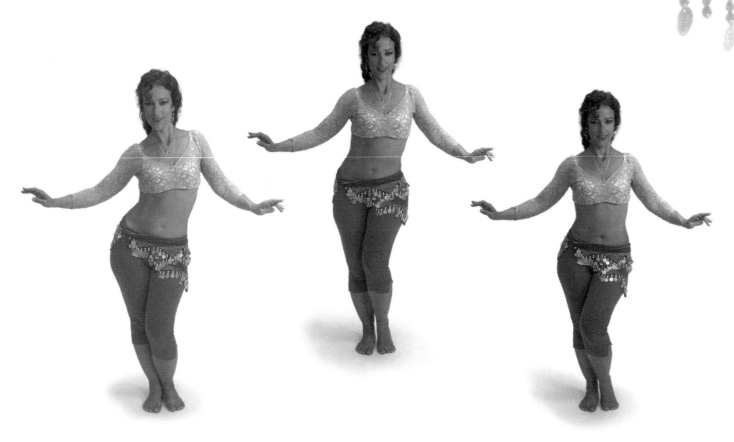

1 With your ankles together, push your right hip out, both feet flat. Tighten the right buttock, causing the fringe or coins on your hipscarf to jump.

2 Keeping your hips slid to the right, lift the left heel and hip up, directly under your ribcage.

3 Keeping your left heel up, drop the left hip. Hold the fourth beat. Don't move! *Then switch sides.*

*Do the Three-Quarters Shimmy 32 times (16 on each side, alternating).*

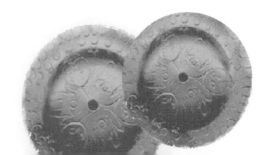

# Medium-Tempo Movements

## Use Medium-Tempo Music

Medium-tempo movements allow the dancer time to breathe since they're not as intense as the slow movements and not as aerobic as the Shimmies.

Movements using **One Hip at a Time** (such as Hip Drops and One-Hip Crescents) improve your balance and look great on the dance floor. Very rhythmic, they are done on the downbeat of the music—the beat you would naturally clap or walk to.

**Traveling Steps** can be done either moving in one direction or in place. What they have in common is that they fill up both the music and the space around you. Traveling steps are easier and less taxing than the other movements. Although they appear lively, they can be considered "resting" steps because they don't require the internal muscle action that other movements do.

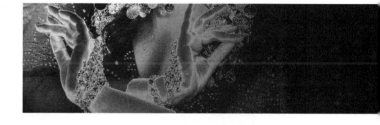

In the olden days,

it was said that a good

belly dancer could keep

her audience riveted

while dancing on

a postage stamp.

# Hip Drop

*Hip Drops will strike a familiar chord in Middle Eastern audiences.*
*A well-timed set of hip drops will inevitably elicit applause.*

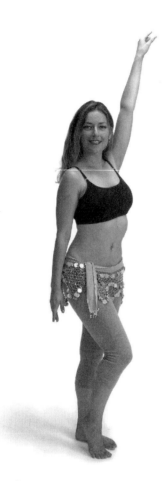
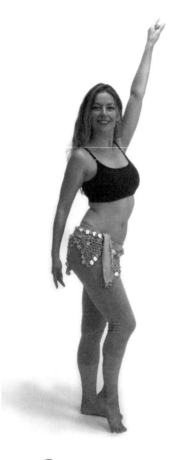
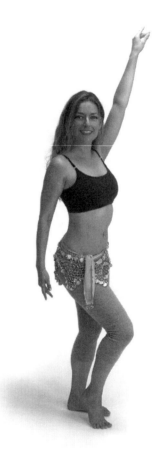

*1* Start with your left foot flat, knee relaxed but not bent. Keeping your knees close together throughout this movement, place your right foot slightly in front of the left, standing on the ball of your right foot. Raise your left arm and let the right arm frame the same-side hip.

*2* Bring your right hip up and drop it down with the beat of the music. By keeping your hips relaxed and bending the knee, your hip will drop naturally.

*Repeat this movement 8 times then switch sides. Do the same sequence again, repeating only 4 times for each hip.*

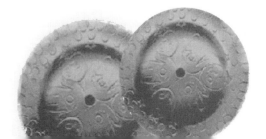

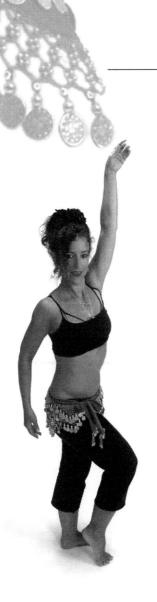

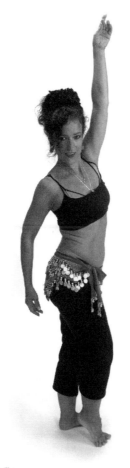

*1* Begin in the same position as the Hip Drop: left foot flat, right foot slightly forward, standing on the ball of the right foot.

*2* Bring your right hip down to start and then lift it up with each beat of the music.

*Repeat 8 times then switch sides. Do the same sequence again, repeating only 4 times for each hip.*

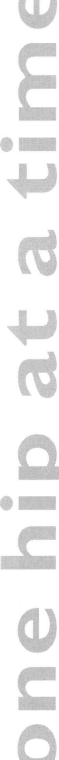

one hip at a time

# One-Hip Twist

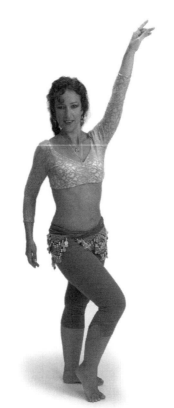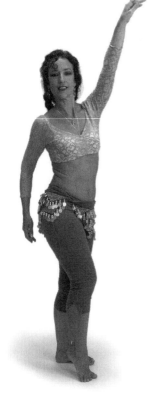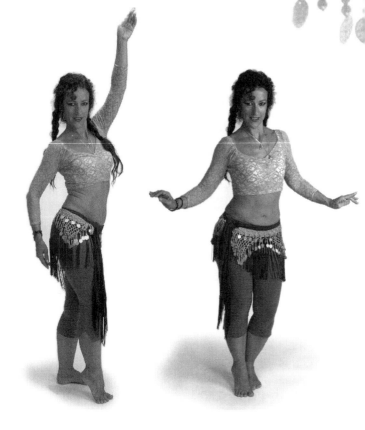

**1** Start in the same position as the Hip Drop or Lift—left foot flat, right foot forward.

**2** Twist the right hip forward with every beat of the music.

*Repeat 8 times then switch sides. Do the same sequence again, repeating only 4 times for each hip. Try also twisting the hip back with the beat instead of forward.*

## variations

**PIVOTING ONE-HIP TWIST:** Keeping the standing leg stationary, pivot as you twist, making a complete circle.

**TWIST ON TOES:** Go up on your toes and keep twisting, but this time, instead of pivoting, travel sideways with the same hip that's twisting.

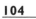

# Hip Drop with a Kick

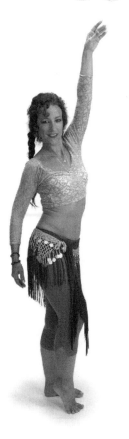

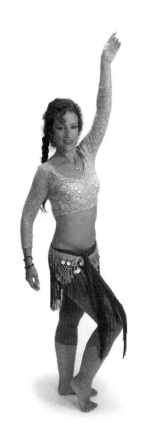

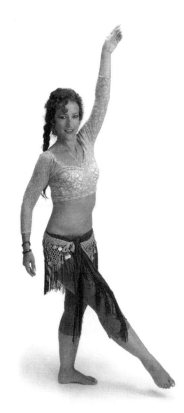

*1* Start in the Hip Drop position—left foot flat, right foot forward.

*2* Drop your right hip once.

*3* Lift your hip, drop your hip again and kick your right foot out. Be delicate and don't kick too high. Repeat: drop, drop and kick, drop, drop and kick. Do your kicks on the second and fourth beats. *Switch sides.*

*Do 4 Hip Drops with a Kick on each side, then repeat for 4 sequences.*

# One-Hip Crescent

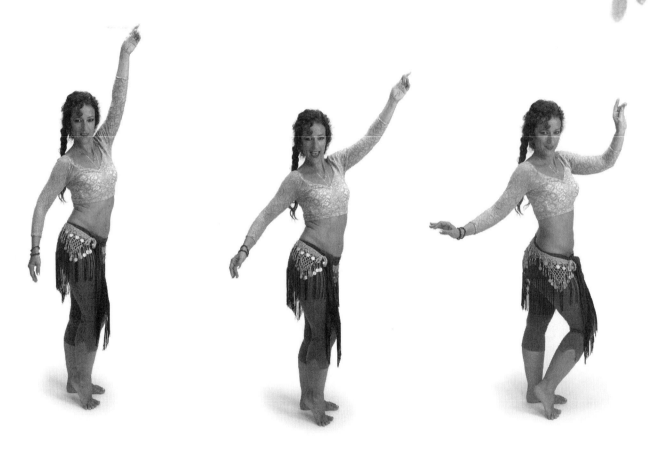

1 Assume the basic Hip Drop position— left foot flat, right foot forward.

2 Lift your right hip in the center.

3 Bring your right hip over and drop it forward.

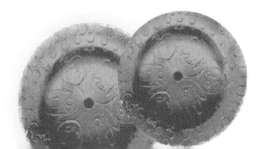

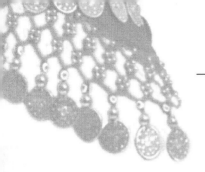

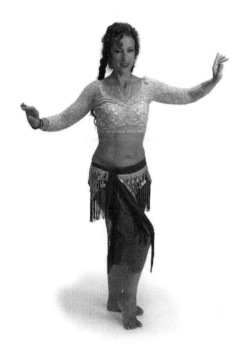

4 Lift the same hip and drop it to the back, bending your right knee each time you drop. *Repeat, alternating forward and back, forward and back. Switch sides.*

*Do 4 One-Hip Crescents on each side, then repeat for 4 sequences.*

# Egyptian Basic

*This elegant movement is a very typical traveling step.*

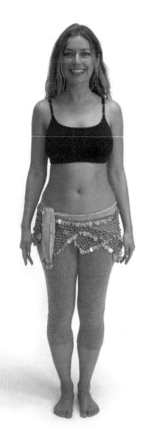

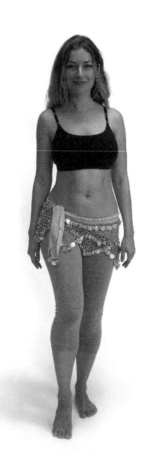

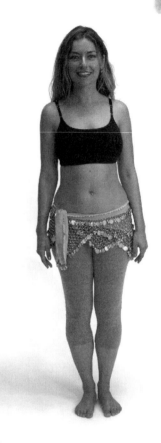

*1* Start with both feet flat.

*2* Keeping the left foot flat, touch the right foot in front with only the ball of the foot.

*3* Return to starting position

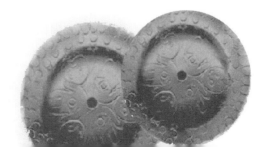

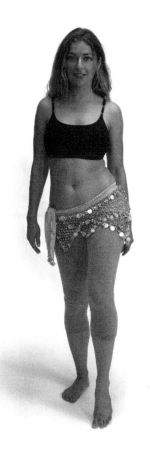

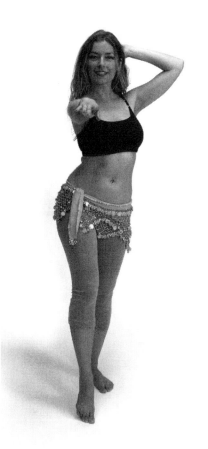

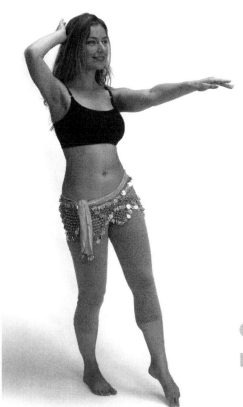

**4** Switch sides. Keeping the right foot flat, touch the left foot in front with only the ball of the foot. Add your hips: Each time the foot touches, the corresponding hip flicks up.

*Do 16 Egyptian Basics.*

Now the arms can be added to give the Egyptian Basic more style: Although they can vary, the most common arm position for the Egyptian Basic is one hand on the forehead or behind the head and the other arm extended straight out.

## In Motion

When you touch with your right foot, extend the right arm and place the left on the head. When you step flat, the arms are in transition. When you touch with your left foot, extend your left arm and place your right hand on the head.

# V-Step

*This is almost the same as an Egyptian Basic except that you cross your feet when you step and touch the ball of your foot out to the side. The catch is that when you cross, the crossing foot has to step flat, otherwise you get stuck and cannot take the next step.*

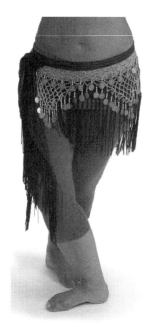 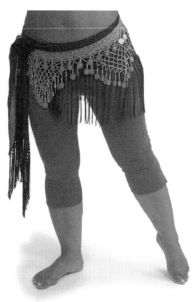 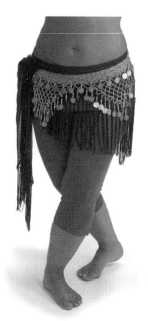 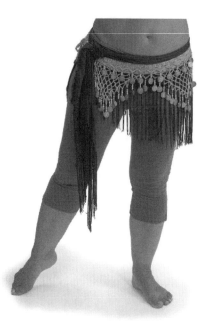

*1* Cross your right foot over the left, placing the right foot flat on the floor.

*2* Bring your left leg out and touch the ball of the left foot to the side.

*3* Cross the left foot over the right, placing it flat on the floor.

*4* Step the right foot out and touch the ball of your right foot to the side. Continue crossing and stepping out. Remember: flat-ball, flat-ball.

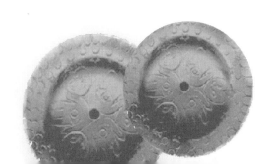

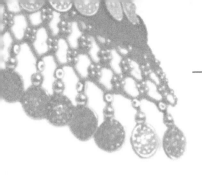

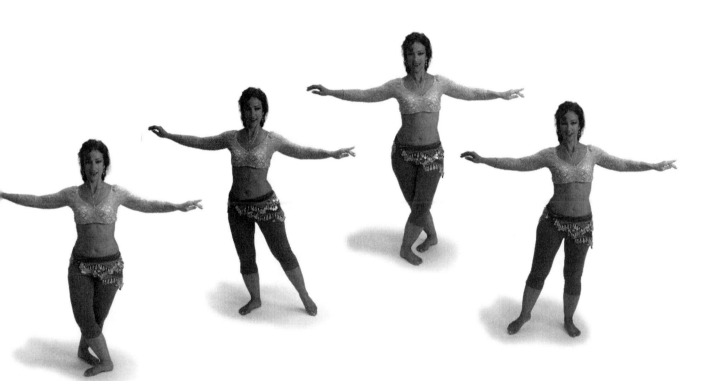

5-8 Add your hips by lifting the corresponding hip each time your foot goes out to the side.

*Do 16 V-Steps.*

# v-Step continued

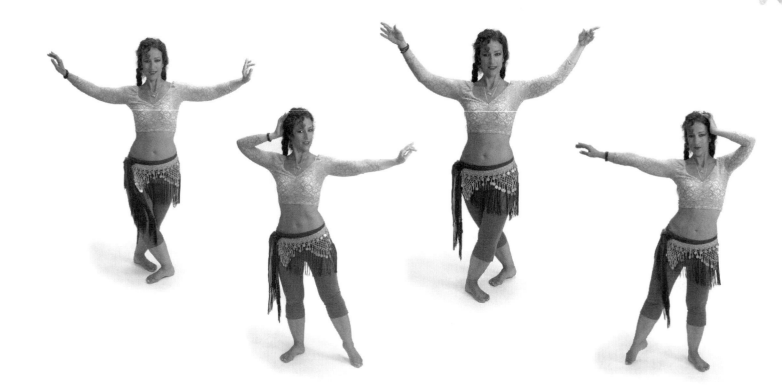

$9$–$12$ Add the arms by placing one hand on the head and extending the other arm out to the side, over the leg that is out.

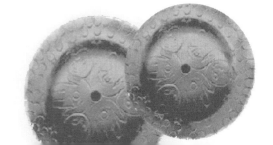

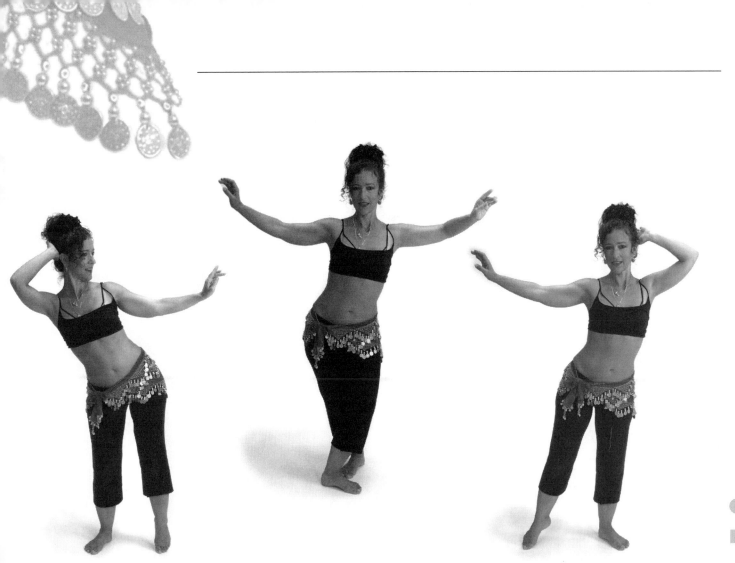

## Putting It Together

Cross the right foot over left, bringing the
left foot out to the side while lifting the hip
and bringing the left arm out, right hand on
the head.

Cross the left foot over right, bringing
the right foot out to the side while lifting
the hip and bringing the right arm out, left
hand to the head.

# Shuffle

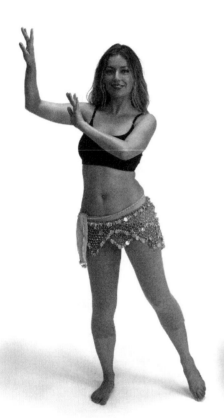 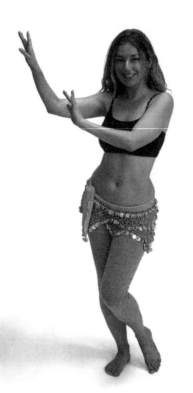 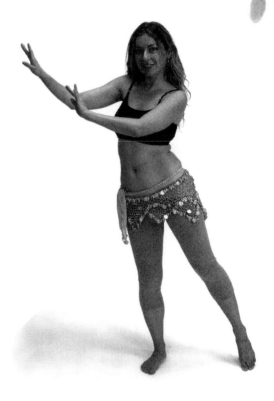

*1* Face the front of the room, feet approximately two feet apart with your right foot flat and weight on the ball of your left foot. The right arm is out and slightly bent, the left arm bent with left hand at the right shoulder.

**TIP:** Keep one foot flat and the other on the ball of the foot at all times. The arms are placed to the side that you are shuffling toward.

*2* Bend your left knee, causing the left hip to drop.

*3* Straighten your left knee, lifting your hip as you Shuffle toward the right. Be sure not to lift either foot off the ground at any time. *Repeat steps 2 and 3. Then switch sides.*

*Shuffle 4 times to the right and 4 times to the left, repeating 8 times in each direction.*

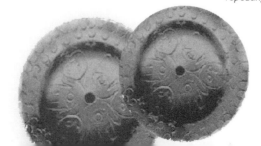

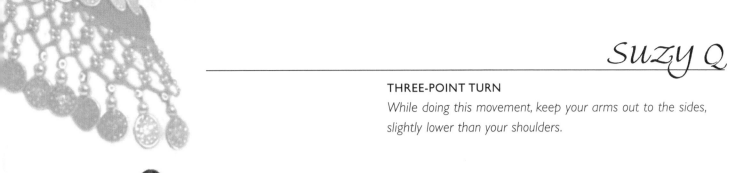

## THREE-POINT TURN

*While doing this movement, keep your arms out to the sides, slightly lower than your shoulders.*

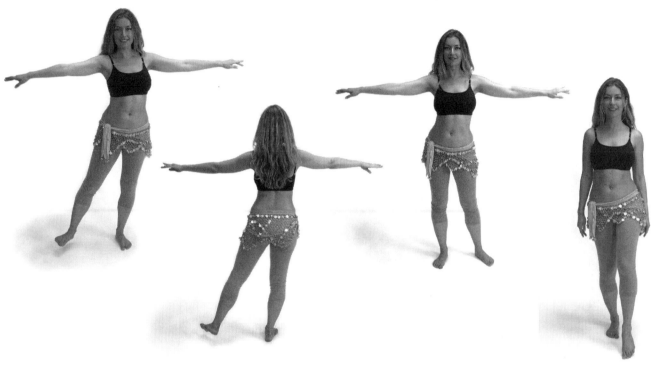

*1* Facing forward, step to the right with your right foot.

*2* Face back by pivoting to the right with your left foot, making a half turn.

*3* Face front again by stepping to the right with the right foot, making another half turn.

*4* This takes up three beats, so on the fourth beat, do an accent: Clap your hands, do a Shoulder Shimmy, or lift and drop your left hip. *Reverse directions.*

*Repeat the Suzy Q 8 times.*

traveling steps

# Scissor Step

*Keeping one foot stationary, the other swings from front to back, creating a rocking motion. The Scissor Step can be done either flat-footed or on the toes, traveling or in place; the arms can be held in a variety of different positions.*

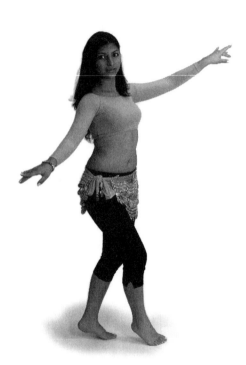

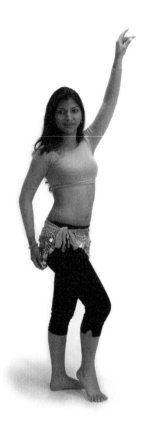

*1* Stand with all your weight on your left leg.

*2* Do the Scissor Step with the right foot, shifting your weight to the right as you step to the front.

*3* Shift your weight to the left as you lift your right foot.

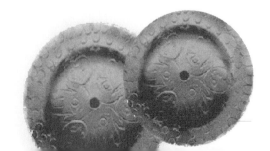

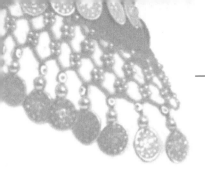

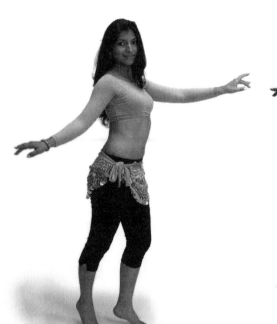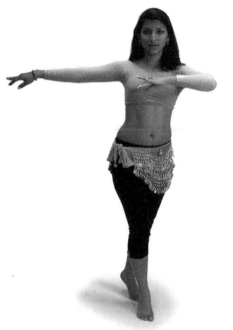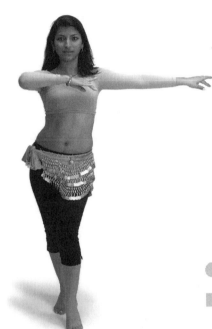

4 Shift your weight to your right once again. *As the right foot goes back, do 16 Scissor Steps with your right. Switch sides.*

The arms can be held in many ways: out to the side as shown in illustrations 1–4; up over your head; or crossing one over your chest and the other out to the side, then switching. Here's how the last one works:

5 Standing on your left foot, step forward with your right, bringing your right arm out and your left arm over the chest.

6 Step back with your right, and bring the right arm over the chest and the left arm out to the side. Keep repeating, switching the arms from side to side. Then try the combination on the other side.

*Repeat the Scissor Step 16 times on each side, using the arm switch.*

117

# skip step

This is a simple step-together-step that can be done either flat-footed or on the toes, traveling forward or traveling backward. Try it on your toes, circling the room. Arms can be done a number of ways, but for now, keep them out to the sides.

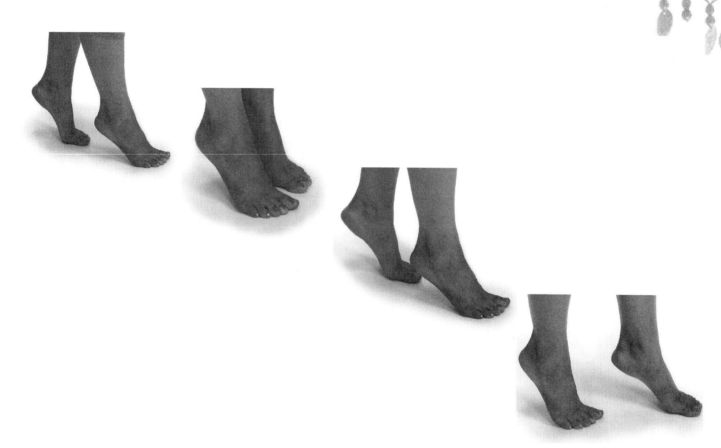

1 Standing on the balls of both feet, bring the right foot forward.

2 Bring the left foot forward to meet it.

3 Then step forward with the right foot again.

4 Switch feet and repeat with the left.

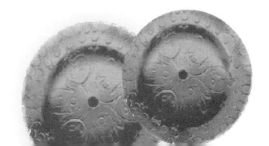

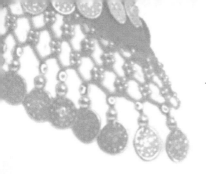

# Arabesque

*This movement is completely different from the Arabesque in ballet. The belly dance Arabesque stays low to the floor, kicking the leg slightly to flick the bottom of your skirt. Your arms should be out to the sides.*

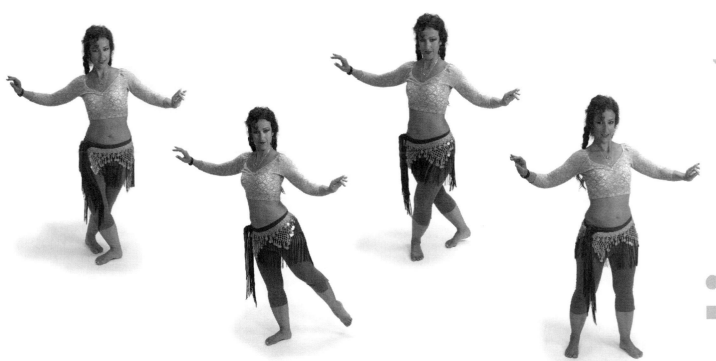

*1* Facing diagonally right, step flat on your right foot.

*2* Kick delicately with your left foot. The left hip faces diagonal while the leg is turned out, knee facing front and toes pointed.

*3* Switching feet, step on the left foot.

*4* Step with your right foot again, continuing in the diagonal to the right. *Switch sides. Alternate the four steps diagonally right, then left, right, and left.*

# Dancing with a Veil

In performance, a traditional Oriental belly dance routine opens with fast, exciting music as the dancer glides with simple steps. Today, belly dancers use veils not only for these fast, gliding entrances, but also to create shapes and swirling illusions with slow songs. It's graceful, showy, and fun.

Assuming that you have enough space in your workout area, Dancing with a Veil makes a perfect relaxing and creative ending for your practice session. Dancing with a Veil also uses your arms, toning and strengthening them, and improves coordination between the feet and arms.

Hold the veil by placing it between your thumb and middle finger, with your arms stretched as far out to the sides as possible.

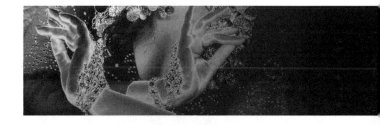

*Get lost in the music*

*and swirling silk—*

*you won't even realize*

*what a head-to-toe workout*

*you are getting.*

# The Veil Entrance

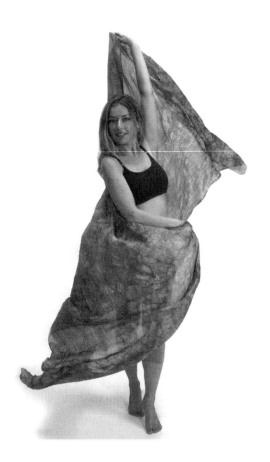

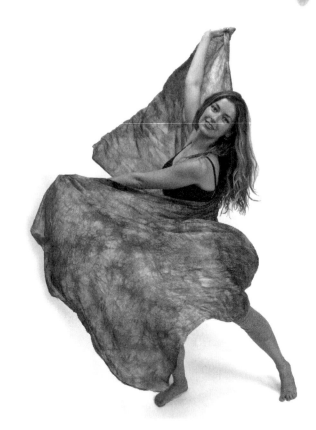

Skip Steps are appropriate traveling steps to use in a Veil Entrance, and we do them with the arms out, up, or switching. I divide them into "Round Arms" and "Straight Arms." As you step-together-step with your right foot, the right arm goes up and the left goes down. Change feet and step-together-step (left, right, left) with your left arm up, right down.

Turns are also appropriate for the opening number. You can turn with your arms up or out to the sides.

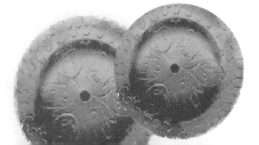

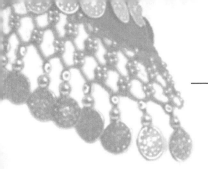

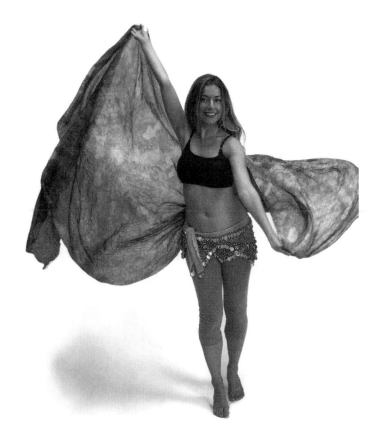

Even a simple walk with the veil billowing behind makes a great intro.

You can add Shoulder Circles, making sure to isolate and only move your shoulders, not your arms or hands.

Arabesques are also very effective for Veil Entrances.

# Slow Dancing with Veil

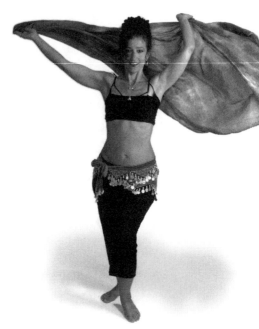

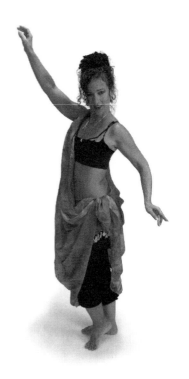

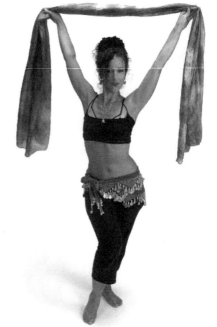

Begin wrapped in your veil. In this case, wrap it like a toga over your right shoulder, with an even amount of fabric in the front and back. Make a ponytail with a corner of the front half and tuck it into the left side of your hip scarf. Make another ponytail with a back corner and tuck it into your left hip.

When you are ready to remove the veil, with your right hand take the front ponytail out first. Then take out the back ponytail with your left hand.

Here are a few cool moves:

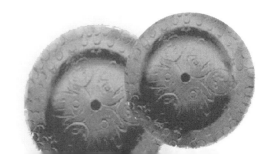

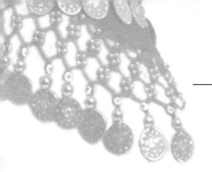

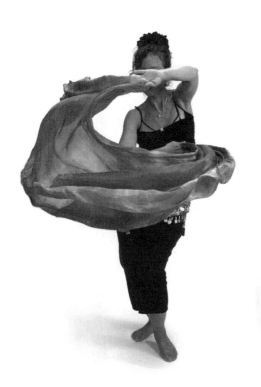

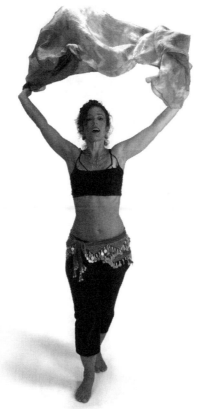

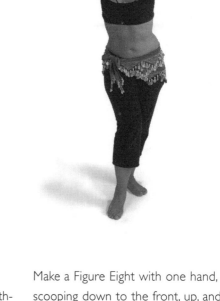

Try twirling for a dramatic effect. With both hands, remove the veil from your neck and lift it overhead. Find the edge of your veil and let the rest unfold. Twirl the veil overhead with one arm at a time. The right arm circles forward and over your head. Then the left hand circles back and overhead. Keep the veil at chest level, not below.

Toss the veil from the front over your head to the back. Put your hands together to lift, and separate them when it is overhead. Let the veil drop behind you. Toss it from the back to front, also bringing your hands together overhead.

Make a Figure Eight with one hand, scooping down to the front, up, and down to the back.

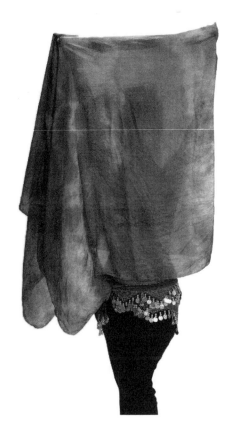

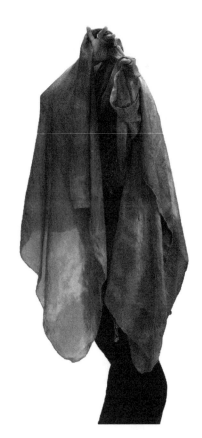

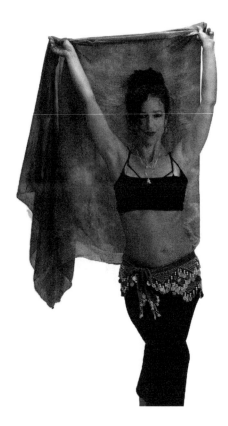

The Envelope is fun and effective. Bring both sides of the veil together, holding them both in your right hand and making sure there is an opening that you can come out of. Slide your left hand to the center of the veil and hold it. You are now inside the Envelope.

Pass your left hand under the right without letting go of any part of the veil. When you open your arms, voila! Like magic, you are outside of the Envelope.

You can re-enter the Envelope by bringing the veil to the front and putting the left arm through the opening, being careful not to let go. Now you are inside again.

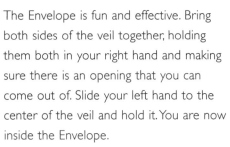

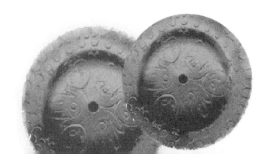

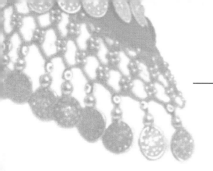

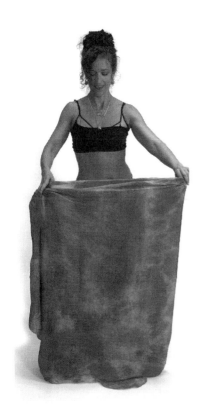

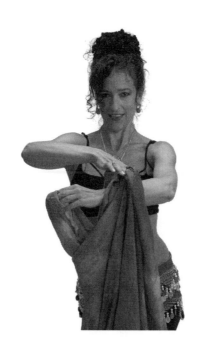

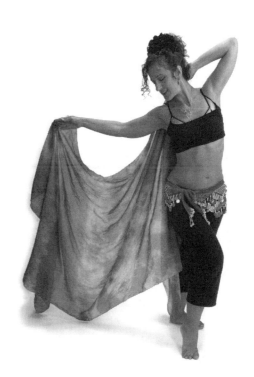

There are many things you can do with the veil, and the most important is to be creative. Practice at home with your own veil every chance you get, not necessarily just during workout sessions. By experimenting, you can come up with new ideas on your own.

# Floorwork

## Use Slow Music

What belly dancers call "floorwork" is dancing on your knees or while lying on the floor. Some say it originated from dancing in tents. In performance, it is usually done to slow, dramatic music in the latter part of a show. I suggest only going on the floor once so as to avoid redundancy. In one of my early student performances, I dropped to the floor with dramatic flourishes five times in 15 minutes. A nice Arabian man gently explained to me that less is more, and I have appreciated the Eastern concept of restraint and subtlety ever since.

Floorwork has been banned in Egypt since the 1950s, and today only the most famous dancers can get by with a few moments on the floor. It can be performed in a suggestive manner that crosses that invisible line between good and bad taste, offending the Egyptian government's deep concern about modesty issues.

Certain costumes are more appropriate for floorwork than others. Tight skirts and high-heeled shoes are awkward. Skimpy skirts with a lot of openings or costumes with cutouts may give the audience more of a show than you intended. Costumes with lots of heavy stones and beads near the knees can be painful to kneel down in. The best costuming for floorwork is a full skirt or harem pants. Both give you a lot of freedom and mobility. Floorwork is especially effective while balancing a sword on your head. (Needless to say, swords are not for novices.)

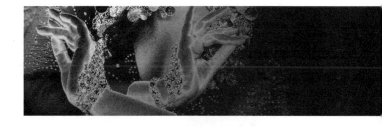

*Tasteful floorwork is another chance to add variety to your dance.*

# Floorwork

There is nothing like floorwork to develop strong thigh muscles. Give floorwork a try using these basic movements you've already learned:

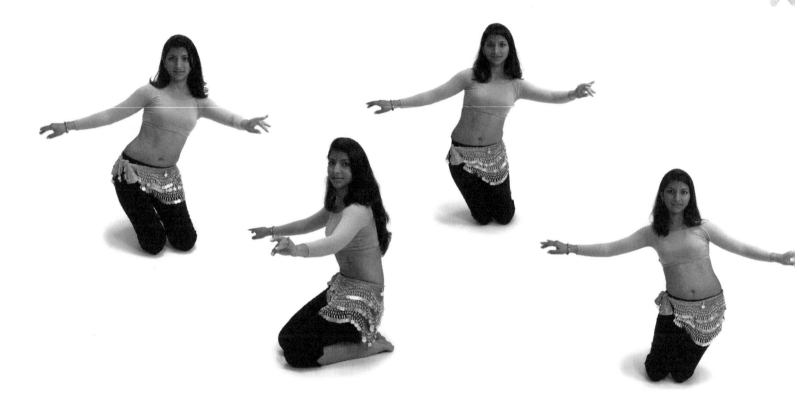

Vertical Figure Eights while kneeling.

Small Hip Circles while kneeling.

Horizontal Figure Eights while kneeling.

Medium Hip Circles from the sitting position to kneeling upright.

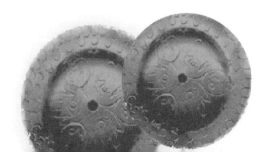

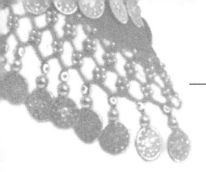

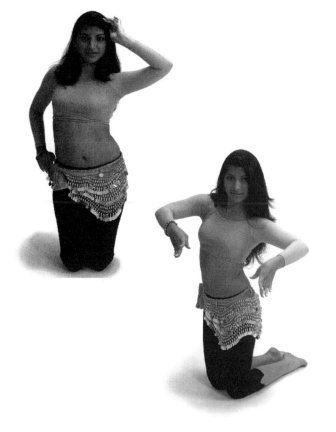

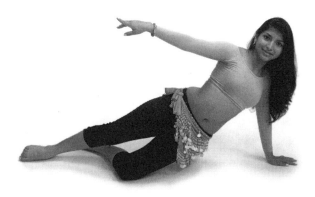

Ribcage Circles while kneeling.     Arm and hand movements while kneeling.

Pelvic Undulations while laying sideways, propped up on one hand.

**TIP:** Floorwork can be hard on the knees, and if yours are delicate, you may want to practice with knee pads.

# *Floorwork* continued

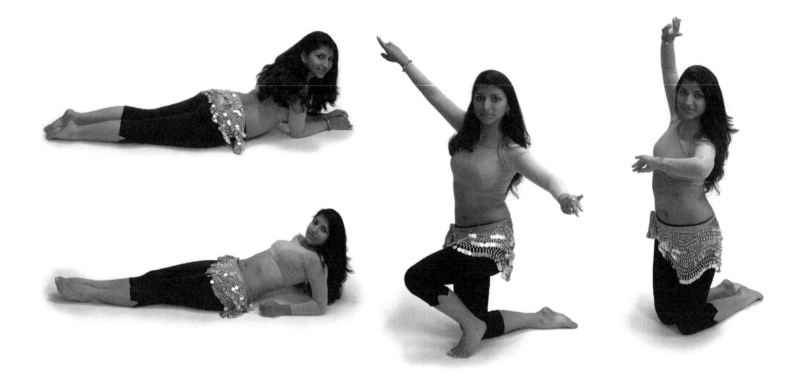

Rolling over, propped first on one elbow and then the other.

Hip drop on one knee.

Walking on your knees.

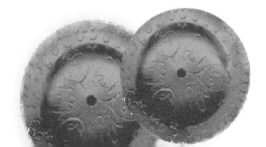

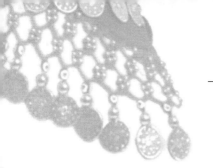

# Backbends

Backbends are not for the timid and you can forgo them if you'd like. If you choose to work up to the backbends, they will give your stomach a workout, stretch your thighs and groin muscles while strengthening your back. Backbends are a beautiful part of belly dancing, but they require strength, flexibility, and lots of practice.

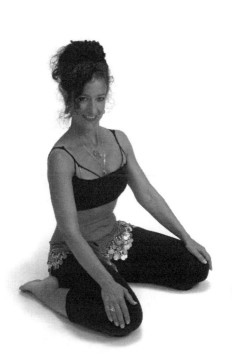 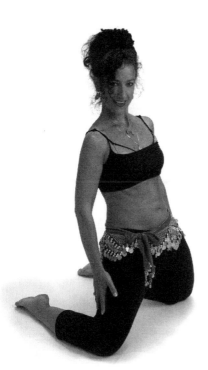 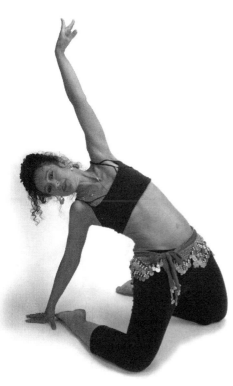

*1* Start by opening your knees and sitting on the floor, butt between your heels.

*2* Gently lift your pelvis up. Push forward and down 10 times to build strength in your thigh muscles. With each push, lean back a little more.

*3* Arch your back and touch one hand to the floor without lowering the pelvis.

floorwork

# Backbends continued

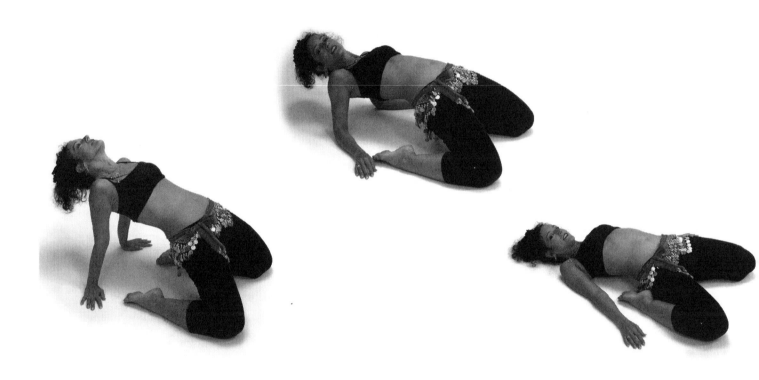

**4** When you're comfortable with this, try touching the floor with both hands, keeping the pelvis up.

**5** Once you find touching the floor with both hands fairly easy (this may take a few days), drop slowly from your hands to your elbows, keeping your pelvis up and your back arched.

**6** After several practice sessions, when you feel more comfortable and confident, drop down to your shoulders (do not touch the floor head-first) then slide flat until your upper body is laying flat on the floor and your hips are also touching the floor. Laying in this position is an excellent stretch—but please work up to this gradually, and stop immediately if any part of your body hurts.

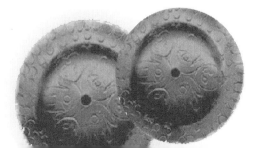

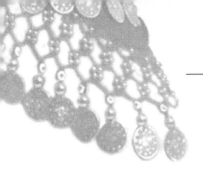

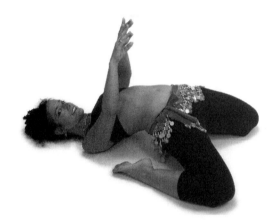

*7* The finishing touch is to achieve the backbend with no hands. If you can do this, the ultimate challenge is to get up the same way you came down. Slide up, lifting first your pelvis, then your upper back, your shoulders, and finally your head.

There are also easier ways to get up that are equally dramatic. Roll over from the backbend into a position laying on one side, propped up on one elbow. Or sweep your body around from the back to side to front and then up.

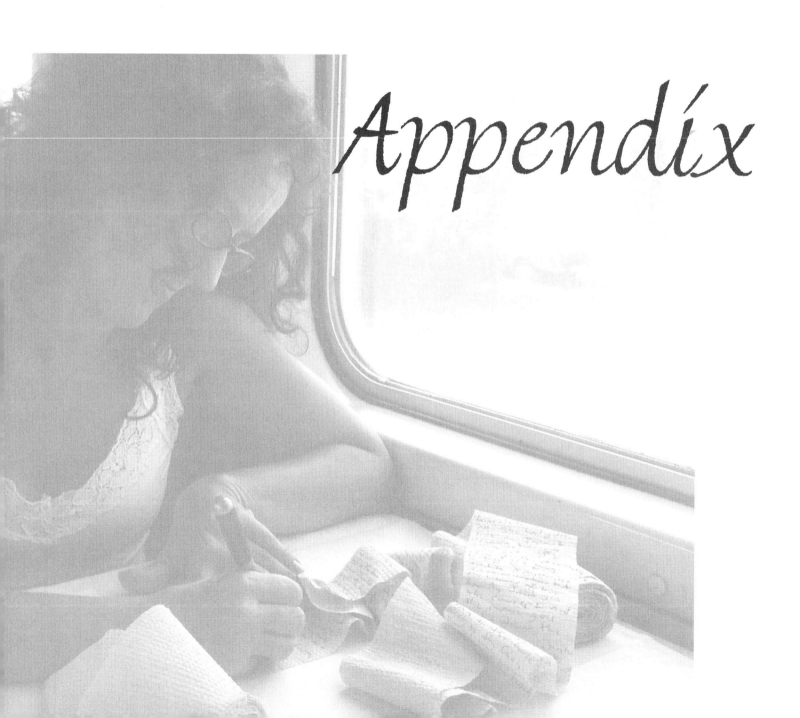

*Appendix*

# what's in a Name?

**B**elly dancers commonly take on Middle Eastern names. You can, too. If you're simply dancing for exercise, this might seem a bit farfetched, but read on . . . you might find a bit of yourself in one of these names. Many more ideas can be found by searching the web for "Arabic names" or "belly dance names."

Most belly dance names are of Arabic origin, though Turkish names are also common, as are Persian and Indian names. Some dancers alter their own names just enough to make them sound exotic. You can also keep your first name and add an exotic-sounding last name. Here are some things to keep in mind when choosing a name:

- What does it mean in Arabic? It might be a wonderful name in one language, but mean something totally ridiculous in another.
- Does another dancer in your area already have that name? Some names are so nice that several professional dancers might have them, but only one dancer per geographical area should take the same name to avoid confusion.
- If you are metaphysically inclined, you might want to find out what number your new name adds up to and ask a numerologist whether the name will be auspicious for you or not.

The following is a brief list of some of the more popular names and what they mean; unless otherwise stated, they are of Arabic origin.

Aasal ~ Honey
Aisha ~ Wife of Mohammed
Amar ~ Moon
Amina ~ Trustworthy and faithful
Amira ~ Princess
Atira ~ Connoisseur of fragrances
Aziza ~ Precious
Azza ~ Strong, bright

Besma ~ Smile
Badawia ~ Bedouin
Dalal ~ Pampered, spoiled (in a good way)
Delilah ~ From "Samson and Delilah"
Dunia ~ The world
Electra (Greek) ~ Shining bright
Esma (Turkish) ~ Brunette
Feiruz ~ Turquoise
Farida ~ Unique, precious
Fatisma ~ Wife of Ali
Ghazala (Persian) ~ Ghazelle
Habibah ~ Beloved
Jalilah ~ Great
Jamila ~ Beautiful
Jawahir ~ Jewels
Johari ~ Jewel
Kadife (Turkish) ~ Velvet
Kamila ~ Perfect, complete
Karima ~ Generous
Khalida ~ Immortal
Latifa ~ Good
Leila or Layla ~ Night
Naima ~ Blessing, happiness
Najla ~ Big eyes
Najma ~ Star
Nazirah ~ Leader, vanguard
Nura or Noor ~ Light
Rashida ~ Intelligent
Sabah ~ Morning
Salome ~ The biblical princess who seduced her stepfather in exchange for the head of John the Baptist (see the opera before taking this name)
Samia ~ Noble
Samira ~ Night-time storyteller
Samra ~ Dark
Shakira ~ Grateful, content
Shahrazad (Persian) or Sheherazade ~ The princess who spun stories to save her life in *1001 Nights*.
Tajah ~ Crown
Yasmin ~ Jasmine

# Resources

## Classes

In addition to using this book, it's important to take classes if they are available. This book, as well as instructional videos, is a valuable learning aid and can guide you step-by-step through daily practice sessions at home between classes. You can also use the workouts in this book to keep up your fitness regimen after completing a series of introductory classes. But neither this book nor a video can give you corrections and feedback that a good teacher will.

Ask around. Look in the Yellow Pages or on the Internet for a studio or school that specializes in Middle Eastern dance. Every city in America has belly dance teachers, though in some places they are not publicized and can be hard to find. Several belly dance publications available by subscription (see "Resources" at the end of this book) contain listings of belly dance teachers in the United States and abroad.

After completing a beginner's course, it's better not to limit yourself to only one teacher, or you're likely to become a carbon copy of her (or his) style. Once you learn the basics, explore and try to learn as much as you can from all the best teachers in town. You should always give credit and respect to your first teacher and to those who have taught you the most, those who have given you support, and those with whom you have studied for any length of time.

Learn as much as you can from as many people as possible—and practice, practice, practice! That is how your own unique style will evolve.

## Instructional Videos

Sooner or later, you'll probably also want to get some belly dance videos or DVDs so you can watch a professional dancer in action as you practice in front of a full-length mirror. There are many on the market; a complete listing can be found in the *All About Belly Dance Video Sourcebook* (see "Resources" in the back of this book). A good video to start with is *Picture Yourself Bellydancing* by yours truly, Tamalyn Dallal. It covers the basic steps and shows how to incorporate them into a routine.

Fortunately, these CDs, videocassettes, and DVDs are a lot easier to get than they used to be. If you live near a book, music, and video store that has a world music section, you'll most likely find what you need there. Otherwise, belly dance music and videos are readily available over the Internet (see "Resources").

## Books

*Serpent of the Nile: Women and Dance in the Arab World* by Wendy Buonaventura and Ibrahim Farrah
  Interlink Publishing Group, 1998
  (A must for every belly dancer's library)

*They Told Me I Couldn't* by Tamalyn Dallal
Talion Publishing, 1997
www.talion.com
(A belly dancer's adventures in Colombia)

*Belly Laughs* by Rod Long
Talion Publishing, 1999
(Belly dancers' adventures with celebrities and other
unusual characters)

*Grandmother's Secrets: The Ancient Rituals and Healing Power
of Belly Dancing* by Rosina-Fawzia B. Al-Rawi
Interlink Publishing Group, 2000
(The history of women's dancing and the story of the
author's coming-of-age in the Arab world.)

# Trade Publications

*Habibi*
PO Box 42018
Eugene, OR 97404
www.habibimagazine.com
Quarterly, $30/year

*Jareeda*
PO Box 680
Sutherlin, OR 97479
www.jareeda.com
jareeda@jareeda.com

*Bennu*
PO Box 20663
Park West Station
New York, NY 10025
www.bellydanceny.com/bennu.html
bennu@aol.com

Caravan
6130 Brook Lane
Acworth, GA 30102
www.caravanmagazine.net
caravan@intergate.net

*Zaghareet!*
PO Box 1809
Elizabeth City, NC 27906
zaghareet.com

# Videos and DVDs

*All About Belly Dance Video Sourcebook*
Donna Carlton, Editor
International Dance Discovery
PO Box 893
Bloomington, IN 47402-0893
(A complete listing of belly dance videos produced
in the United States, updated annually)

Ramzy Music International
11693 San Vicente Boulevard #112B
Los Angeles, CA 90049
(818) 952-6143
www.jannermedia.net
(Vintage Egyptian videos)

Mid-Eastern Dance Exchange
350 Lincoln Road #505
Miami Beach, FL 33139
(305) 538-1608
www.emerald-dreams.com

Instructional videos by Tamalyn Dallal:
Picture Yourself Bellydancing (beginners)
Serious Bellydance (intermediate/advanced)
Also available are several concert videos featuring Tamalyn Dallal, her dance company, and guest performers

Bellydance Superstars
www.bellydancesuperstars.com
Instructional and performance DVDs

## Other Suppliers

Saroyan Mastercrafts
PO Box 2056
Riverside, CA 92516
(909) 783-2050
www.saroyanzils.com
(Fine cymbals, swords, music)

Mideast Manufacturing
7694 Progress Circle
West Melbourne, FL 32904
(407) 724-1477
(Drums and other Middle Eastern musical instruments)
Audrena's International Bazaar
PO Box 26
Chicago Ridge, IL 60415
800-327-3406
audrena.com
(Costumes, accessories, music)

Dahlal International
800-745-6432
www.dahlal.com
(Costumes, accessories, music, videos)

Turquoise International
22830 Califa Street
Woodland Hills, CA 91367
818-999-5542 or 800-548-9422
(costumes, veils, accessories, cymbals, music, videos)

## Websites

www.beledy.net (Florida listings)
www.bhuz.com (nationwide listings)
www.zaghareet.com (worldwide listings)
www.gildedserpent.com (e-zine)
www.ameltafsout.com (lots of history)
www.emerald-dreams.com (Mid Eastern Dance Exchange website)
www.tamalyndallal.com (my site)

## Belly Dance Festivals

Rakkasah
sponsored by Shukriya
1564-A Fitzgerald Drive, Suite 124
Pinole, CA 94564
(510) 724-0214
www.rakkasah.com
(One of the world's largest belly dance festivals; lasts nine days in mid-March, with a smaller version in New Jersey in October)

Utah Annual Bellydance Festival
sponsored by Yasmina and Jason Roque
PO Box 52027
Salt Lake City, UT 84125
(801) 486-7780
www.kismetdance.com
(August)

Music and Dance Camp
3244 Overland Avenue #1
Los Angeles, CA 90034
(310) 838-5471
www.middleeastcamp.com
joshkun@middleeastcamp.com
(Mendocino, CA in August)

Ahlan Wa Hassan
Mme. Raqia Hassan
raqiahassan@hotmail.com or raqia_festival@msn.com
www.raqiahassan.net
(Cairo, Egypt—June/July)

# Index

## ABOUT THE AUTHOR

TAMALYN DALLAL (born Tamalyn Harris in the mountains of Colorado) began belly dancing as a teenager in 1976. In 1990 she founded the Mid Eastern Dance Exchange, a nonprofit arts organization in Miami Beach, Florida, where for the past 14 years she has worked as an instructor, performer, choreographer, and producer of many major live dance shows, including the annual Orientalia festival.

Ms. Dallal was one of the original "Bellydance Superstars" on the CD and DVD from Ark 21 Records. She was named Ms. America of Belly Dance and Miss World of Belly Dance in 1995. She has performed for such celebrities and dignitaries as Robert De Niro, Madonna, James Brown, The Jacksons, Sean Connery, King Abdullah of Jordan, the Saudi royal family, and President Francisco Flores of El Salvador. She has danced in the Orange Bowl parade, choreographed and performed in a dance segment of the Super Bowl halftime show, and produced the series "Belly Dance" for PBS television. Her career has taken her to more than 30 countries, including Egypt, Turkey, Tunisia, Morocco, India, Mexico, Belize, Honduras, Colombia, Brazil, Argentina, Venezuela, Chile, Bolivia, Curacao, Aruba, Haiti, the Dominican Republic, Puerto Rico, the Bahamas, Switzerland, Italy, Bulgaria, Romania, and Japan. In 2004 she turned over the directorship of the Mid Eastern Dance Exchange in order to spend more time traveling to teach workshops, perform, and research dances.

## ABOUT THE PHOTOGRAPHER

Born in Brooklyn, New York, and raised in Latin America, DENISE J. MARINO opened her vision to many different cultures at an early age. With her camera, she started capturing colorful images from all over the world. Her collection of photographic images includes documentation of social functions, theatrical performances, portraits, and artistic images. She has won many awards and been extensively published in various magazines, including *Geomundo* magazine and *Donde*. With the emergence of digital photography, her first two experiences were photographing Japan and Cuba. She is currently dedicating her talent to one of the most sensual and vibrant forms of art: belly dancing. Her passion for that art has led her to experience the dance itself and find out that every part of the body is a work of art.